Genevieve

TALKI

Used This a non text book resource when doing a communication paper —

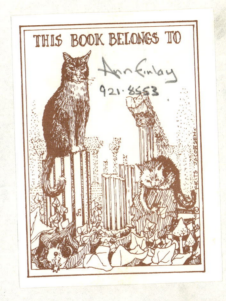

But I'm sure that your class at *that* school will be much more 'informed' & different (changed) attitudes towards "patients"
Also - British Approach!
   But might give some laughs + ideas.

TALKING WITH PATIENTS

Talking with Patients

– *a guide to good practice* –

James Calnan FRCS FRCP

*Emeritus Professor of Plastic & Reconstructive Surgery,
University of London, at the Royal Postgraduate Medical School,
Consultant Surgeon Hammersmith Hospital, London*

Cartoons by James

William Heinemann Medical Books
London

DISCLAIMER

Without disrespect, I have used the male pronoun throughout. I realise that my writing is for both sexes, but to indicate this continually in English is clumsy.

ISBN 0-433-05013-6
First published 1983
Reprinted 1984

© James Calnan 1983

Phototypeset by Tradespools Ltd, Frome, Somerset
and printed and bound in Great Britain by
Biddles Ltd, Guildford and King's Lynn

Contents

1.	**Introduction**	1
	Attitudes	2
	Performance and principles	5
	Profession and professionalism	6
	Improvements	7
	Six important abilities	11
2.	**Communication**	14
	Twelve principles	14
	Communication and the patient	27
	The significance of good spoken communication	30
3.	**Conversation**	32
	Ten principles	34
	Ten aims	35
	Seven golden rules in talking medicine	40
	Humour	43
	Mannerisms	45
4.	**The consultation or interview**	48
	The skill of interviewing	49
	Successful interviewing	52
	Questions	55
	Listening	57
	Some answers	60
5.	**Special people, special occasions**	63
	The deaf	63
	The blind	64
	The speechless	65
	Children and parents	66
	Talking with relatives	67
	Foreigners	69
	Teaching with patients	72
	Research	74
	Consent	76

6.	Talking about diagnosis and prognosis	81
	Explaining the diagnosis	82
	Five useful guides	84
	Why must the patient know the diagnosis?	85
	Consequences of a diagnosis	85
	Prognosis	87
	How to reassure the patient	89
	Expectation	91
	The technique of explanation	93

7.	Talking about treatment	95
	Medical treatment	97
	Compliance	97
	Surgical treatment	102

8.	The fatal illness	111
	Talking about dying	112
	Planning your talk	114
	The patient's attitude to his diagnosis	119
	Comfort	122
	Talking with the bereaved	124
	Talking with staff	126

9.	Complaints and criticism	128
	Common causes for complaints	128
	Understanding complaints	130
	Dealing with complaints	133

References and further reading	138

Index	145

1
Introduction

*'Life is short, the art long, timing is exact, experience
treacherous, judgement difficult.'*

Hippocrates

The trouble about writing a book is this: no-one can write about talking with patients and get it right because reality is always more complex than any author can express. Yet the author's duty remains quite clear: to bring such order as he can perceive into the chaos of available fact. So much for writing, what about talking?

Talking with patients is an endless task, but rewarding if a few simple techniques are learnt, understood and practised. But practising talking is not enough. You must believe passionately that it is important to talk with that particular patient. Eventually you will develop a conscience which says every time: 'Have I said enough or too much, could I have spoken more kindly, listened more carefully?' The trouble with modern medicine is that it is so easy to give tablets which will cure that there is no obvious need to talk. Curative treatment says it all, silently and effectively.

When you are learning a skill, once the ground rules and general disciplines become second nature, you can explore and experiment. Understand first that talk is fundamentally a simple process which should come naturally, but can the ability to talk with patients be acquired? Yes, I am sure of that, and we can do better than the mediocrity that passes for communication today. In matters of life and death – medicine and nursing deal with both – communication should be above mere competence; it should be excellent. We grumble about patients' non-compliance in treatment, when the fault lies in ourselves. We expect cooperation but are unable to define it. Yet the techniques of good communication, of talking with patients, can be taught and learnt and these skills put into daily practice.

2   *Talking with Patients*

Talking with patients is perhaps the most important aspect of medicine for nurses and doctors because it is the most reliable form of communication. When a patient refers to a 'good doctor' or 'good nurse' he often means someone to whom he can talk easily. In many medical conditions talking is therapeutic. Balint (1957) has pointed out that the most potent drug in medical practice is the doctor himself. This applies equally to the nurse. Talent for talking is mandatory for both yet there is no mystique involved, and no-one should wonder what is so special about talking with patients. The mystery is why people do it badly. Asher (1972) wrote 'The way we deal with our patients, and especially how we talk to them, is about the most important part of our trade; but can it be taught?' He answered his own question with a doubtful 'no', although admitting that much can be learnt by experience and by watching great doctors handling their patients, 'but it cannot be taught like pharmacology'. I agree. Pharmacology is a more exact technology, based on the science of chemistry, whereas human relationships are less easy to define and there are many permutations between doctor, nurse and patient.

Talking is not a purely personal thing, however. It is true that there are areas of option and that, within these areas, we can each develop our individual style. But behind these options lie basic principles that can be taught in a methodical manner. This book sets out to teach those principles and to indicate some of the options.

ATTITUDES

Real attitudes show. If you cannot continue to meet your patients in a genuinely friendly, even-tempered way, then change your job. You can't fake attitudes; if you try to fake them, patients will come away with a vague feeling of uneasiness, some suspicion, and a certain distaste which may determine permanently their opinion of you. The forced smile serves no purpose, because patients need genuine friendliness, genuine sympathy. The false is spotted quickly, even by your own colleagues.

The first contact with your patient should be a smile, the second touch, the third a question 'What can I do for you?' By

Introduction 3

using the three senses of sight, touch and speech by way of greeting, the patient will realise that you are prepared to give him warm, courteous attention, and he will react favourably.

The proper attitude calls for an awareness of patients, the human context of medicine, not just their diseases. You have to go deeper. You have to talk with the patient outside the line of duty.

Geoffrey Ashe (1979) gave this advice to would-be writers: 'This, then, is the first principle of all. Be conscious of the society around you, and cultivate the right attitude towards it. Maintain awareness, even when you think there's nothing exciting to be aware of. Maintain respect, even when you think there's nothing much to respect.' The same advice should be heeded by talkers. Awareness, attitude and respect: these three determine how you talk with patients.

Few people learn the skill of talking naturally to patients unless they have to, and we do have to. A sense of compulsion is important. So the advice is to try to develop an exceptional ability in talking well and then, if you wish to become outstanding, develop an uncanny deductive skill. To obtain these virtues requires a lot of practice, experience, perception, and the ability to listen and to reason with yourself and your patient; it is not impossible, but it is a demanding and constant

---

1.1 The emotional stress of talking

1. Increased pulse and respiration rate.

2. Changes occur in electrocardiogram tracings.

3. Increased plasma catecholamines.

4. Increased plasma free fatty acids.

5. Dry mouth.

6. Sweating.

7. Increased blood sugar level.

8. Jerky speech.

9. Abnormal body movements.

10. Forgetfulness.

---

4   Talking with Patients

task. The reward is a precious thing. For not only will you become a good clinician you will also become a very able diagnostician, a person to be consulted by your own colleagues – surely the highest accolade, and eminently satisfying.

There are competent doctors and nurses who, while excellent at their job, are completely unable to speak tactfully; they manage unintentionally to provoke discontent among patients and colleagues. They are well-meaning but awkward (and sometimes quite offensive) in dealing with other people; they seem to lack feeling for the sensitivities of others; they fail to recognise that their actions appear to be selfish and demanding, which they sometimes are; and they are unable to do anything to correct the bad impression they make, a sort of colour blindness, even when these defects in character are gently pointed out. What can be done for these unfortunates? After years of experience, I suspect very little. Perhaps they should be encouraged to divert their energies to fields where direct contact with patients can be avoided, such as general administration or laboratory work. Some, of course, do improve themselves by persistent hard work and turn out to be the best of speakers.

The vast majority communicate well but could do better. Doctors and nurses formulate their own system of behaviour in talking to patients, from a wide range of previous experiences: from their teachers in hospital, from their own family doctor, from a relative in medicine, or worst of all from a few television fantasies. The skill is something which doctors and nurses are expected to pick up as they progress through training, possibly because of the difficulty assumed in deciding what has to be learned.

1.2 Three forms of talking

1. Narration: to tell a story. Events are arranged in a time sequence.

2. Exposition: to explain why, how, what, where, who and when. It is the commonest form of talk with patients.

3. Argument: to persuade, so uses logic, premises, examples.

Introduction 5

PERFORMANCE AND PRINCIPLES

What the practising nurse and doctor need is skill rather than knowledge in talking to patients. The role of an instructor is merely to act as a guide. This book is no more than a guide for the learner to find out things for himself, but to find out does require effort and interest. The reward of acquiring a useful skill far outweighs the effort required. The learner will discover the principles and relationships of effective communication and will develop an understanding of their implications.

Management of patients in hospital and general practice is becoming increasingly the art of persuasion and participation. Hence doctors and nurses of the future will have to improve their powers of persuasion and flexibility in talking. Management by consent rather than management by coercion is commonly called salesmanship. In the past, medical salesmanship has been a poor effort. We have dismally failed to persuade people to help themselves to prevent all those illnesses directly attributable to social excesses such as smoking, taking alcohol, and physical inertia. Persuasion is not the same as manipulation; persuasion rests on reason, willingness, belief and self-conviction. Manipulation is like using antibiotics to treat the chronic bronchitis from excessive smoking, instead of a more logical and persuasive conversation with advice on personal habits.

Anyone's performance in a given job is a function of three different complexes – ability, energy, motivation – which are all personal characteristics. There is little evidence that any of them, in the adult, can be altered by training or exhortation. So we all have to make the best of our natural traits by self-discipline and practice.

The principles of communication in medicine are now well known; the difficulty is to transfer them to daily clinical practice, to teach them so that their value will be recognised and appreciated. It must be admitted that a busy, crowded and under-staffed out-patient clinic (in hospital or general practice) is not the ideal place for developing the skills of interviewing. Even so, every nurse and doctor acts as a public relations officer for his place of work, at least in the eyes of the patient. Hence

6   *Talking with Patients*

there is a duty to acquire the skills of talking. The title 'Talking with Patients' has been used deliberately to emphasise the art and skills required in the everyday life of medical students, junior doctors and nurses; particularly nurses, who have the greater opportunity to speak with a patient.

1.3 The good talker

1. Is sensitive to his listener.
2. Strives to make the other respond.
3. Looks interested.
4. Always allows the other to speak when he wishes.
5. Follows the lead indicated by another.
6. Is entertaining, has humour.
7. Uses language with feeling and sensitivity.
8. Discovers topics which interest the other.
9. Is a good listener.
10. Knows when to stop.

PROFESSION AND PROFESSIONALISM

Talking with patients and explaining things is the firm responsibility of the doctor and nurse looking after the patient. Failure to do so is 'knowingly to do harm'. According to psychologists and behavioural therapists we are expected to have insight into all our patients' problems. We are expected to have empathy and an understanding of the individual's psychological needs. This is absurd. It means that the doctor and nurse are expected to be omniscient. Most medical people find it hard enough to know all they need to know about their own immediate area of expertise, be it surgery, medicine or nursing. To expect everyone to have charisma, whatever that might mean, is an absurdity because this particular quality is reserved for the few.

A more practical suggestion is that doctors and nurses should know more than they do about human beings and about themselves. There has to be mutual respect between patient,

Introduction 7

nurse and doctor. The integrity of the nurse and doctor lies in their subordination to the requirements of a common task, the patient's welfare: in both there is need for authority but on different grounds. All need the skills of good communication for without them there is little professionalism in the task of belonging to a profession. This book tries to set out the principles of good communication in medicine between one person and another, to offer a guide to effective practice.

It is the duty of the doctor and nurse not to conceal reality, not to cause social disruption, and not to prevent understanding. Failure in any one of these is a grievous social harm. And for the individual patient? In truth, professional help does not consist in playing God with the patient, but in placing the professional's knowledge and skill at the disposal of the patient. The doctor or nurse may advise, explain, persuade, describe, but never demand although he does have to talk with the patient in language that is simple, direct and understandable.

Nurses and doctors are trained in hospital and that is where they must learn the skills of talking with patients. When they leave hospital the setting for practice may change, but the skill should remain. My remarks are therefore hospital based, but talking is an essential part of medicine and nursing wherever they are practised.

1.4 The English we use depends on

1. Social background.
2. Education level.
3. Age.
4. Geographical location.
5. The occasion.
6. The listener.

IMPROVEMENTS

How can talking with patients be improved? First by recognising that there is a problem and that sometimes patients do complain that they have not been told the diagnosis and

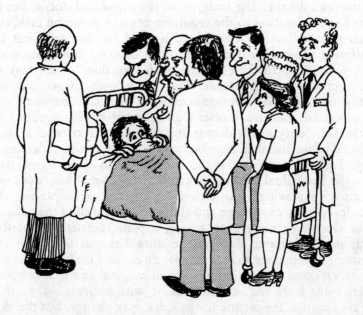

treatment of their disease when in fact they have. Often the more intelligent and knowledgeable the patient, the greater the grouse. Who is to blame? It seems to me that there are faults on both sides. The patient only consults a doctor when he is ill; he is rightly anxious and not as receptive as he might be to the spoken word. In the strange environment of a consulting room, besides listening to words he may not fully understand, he is worrying about his job, his family and his own future. When he leaves and has time to think, a host of questions occur to him, but there is no-one to answer them, which worries him even more.

In hospital, for investigations or treatment, the situation worsens: he is now in an alien environment where routine and rules govern the day and his main source of information may only be the patient in the next bed. The doctor and nurse on the other hand, used to every-day medical terms and their own routine, tend to assume that the patient will pick up the essentials quickly; they have many patients to look after and little time to spend talking with one. As a result, the patient gets the idea that they are arrogant and uncaring which is usually untrue. In hospital, nurses have a great deal of work to do

Introduction 9

within a specified time and so cannot always stop to chat. The patient is hungry for conversation and companionship, comfort and reassurance; he is lonely and his pride is hurt by illness; his mind and body are equally afflicted yet no-one seems to care. Above all else he wants someone to talk with.

Perhaps it is not so much a lack of communication as a lack of understanding on both sides. After all, in the consulting room there is personal confrontation of one patient with one doctor, surely the most favourable condition for excellent communication. Yet even here the effective exchange of knowledge may fail.

Of course the good talker is a bit of an actor too. He is sensitive to his audience (the patient), sensitive of his personal technique and always looking for something better, sensitive to the patient's needs and changing state. He is an artist. Art, says the dictionary, is skill as a result of knowledge and practice. That's all? Yes, that's all. Whenever one makes or performs something with skill, and with concern for its excellence, one is an artist. Hence one, anyone, can become an artist in talking with patients. To quote one famous aside: 'The artist is not a special kind of man, but every man is a special kind of artist.'

Doctors and nurses have certain obligations, duties and privileges. The privileges may narrow but the standards must not; these are the standards of behaviour, rectitude, integrity, dress, knowledge and practice. In patient care only the best is good enough – until something better comes along.

The following dozen items are surely important.

● Never refuse to see or talk with a patient when asked to do so.

● Act in a dignified way, without being pompous, but be friendly.

● Be sensitive to the patient's worries and illness.

● Realise that information extracted from the patient is confidential and may be extremely personal.

● Speak with confidence and authority, which mainly comes from knowledge and previous experience.

● Never be afraid to say that you don't know, and always to follow this with the promise to find someone who does know, who can help and whom you can recommend with confidence from personal knowledge.

10 Talking with Patients

● Always make it clear to the patient, directly or indirectly, that you have a strict code of conduct and recognised ethical standards.

● Speak clearly, concisely and with patience. The doctor and nurse must define what they mean, simply because medical terms are often clichés and the layman may be misled if technical words are not explained at the time. If a patient does not understand the meaning of a word he will often ask other lay people who may give a totally incorrect definition.

● Patients' questions should be answered truthfully. When a patient asks a question it should be assumed that he wants to know the answer. Admittedly this is not always so, but is in general true. It is therefore presumptuous of the doctor to decide that a patient should be spared the truth about himself if he asks for it, unless there is good reason to believe the contrary. Being truthful is not the same as being blunt.

● The patient must be left with something to look forward to, and even the most dreadful prognosis need not be given without the comfort of hope for the few remaining days. The doctor must give a commitment to continue care, by offering the patient with a terminal illness a future clinic appointment or some other indication that he intends to continue symptomatic treatment.

● When the seriously ill or terminal patient in hospital is sedated it is kinder to wake him up during a ward round if only to exchange a few words. If the patient is allowed to sleep through the ward round his subsequent sense of rejection (by being overlooked or ignored) may be more damaging to his morale than waking him up. Alternatively, make a point of returning to see him alone a few hours later and explain why.

● Physical contact is important. A hand on the arm or shoulder concentrates mental contact so that the patient feels reassured and not entirely alone in the world. For the old, the lonely and very ill this simple action can be more effective than words.

In talking there is only one standard – the best. This is not the same as equality because some patients require more informa-

Introduction 11

tion and reassurance more often than others. 'We'll get you well' suffices for the desperately ill: but when they recover, explanations are in order and essential. Many visits with a little information at a time are better than too much at one time.

Quality is another matter. Archie Cochrane (1976) put it this way: 'We all recognise quality when we see it and particularly when we receive it. In "cure" the outcome plays an important part in determining quality, but it is certainly not the whole story. The really important factors are kindliness and ability to communicate on the part of all the members of the medical team. In "care" of course the latter two become very much more important.' Medicine is often described as a vocation, that is professing special learning and applying it to the affairs of others. The practice of the art of medicine, for the benefit of patients and not for oneself, carries a spiritual message of dedication to the patient's welfare. Norbet Wiener, describing the independent scientist, suggested that he should have 'a consecration which comes entirely from within himself: a vocation which demands the possibility of supreme self-sacrifice'. A high ideal, fortunately not often put to the test.

SIX IMPORTANT ABILITIES

The personal touch counts greatly, so you have to be on the spot to explain to each and everyone. Although there is no agreement on the exact personal characteristics that assure a doctor or a nurse of success in talking with patients, here are six valuable qualities that seem to be important.

● Deftness in handling people: this is not the same as 'getting along with people'. The able talker will enjoy being with people, and have the knack of being liked. Managing patients is more than that: the deft will be better than average at sizing up the patient, will inspire loyalty in his subordinates, delegate work smoothly, reprimand in private and never in public, and come to decisions quickly.

● The ability to marshall the essential facts and to solve the

12 Talking with Patients

patient's problem. The man with a competent mind does not necessarily have a high intelligence quotient, but he does need good judgement which is less easy to measure than intelligence; he has the ability to immerse all his thoughts in the problem to hand; he has the capacity to get to the heart of the matter and then come up with alternative solutions, for he will not get lost in detail nor be bogged down in trivia. Thus an orderly mind and good judgement involve several skills – of analysis, assessment, and integration.

● The ability to communicate and originate new ideas. The value of the knack of communicating equally well with patients and with fellow professionals (and other professions for that matter) should never be underestimated. One valuable asset, which can be acquired easily in your spare time, is a large and exact English vocabulary. Another is a large pad of scrap paper on which you can illustrate what you mean, a do-it-yourself audio-visual aid to understanding, to capture the eye while working on the ear.

● The skill to respond to provocation objectively and effectively. This means keeping personal feelings out of crises, by maintaining an emotional detachment with coolness. For some, this is very difficult. Provocation creates anxiety in all of us, but it is the manner of our response that matters. Medical emergencies, things that go wrong, bureaucratic stupidities, complaints and frustrations are all provocative; some galvanise us into action, others freeze us into immobility.

● The ability to enjoy patient care: the important word is enjoy. The man who enjoys responsibility will enjoy the satisfaction of a job well done, and he will be recognised by the patient as accountable for all his actions and decisions. He will thus engender trust.

● The ability to create confidence: the successful nurse or doctor will know where he is going, exactly what he is doing and why, and will convey that impression to the patient. Faith in your own judgement (another mark of leadership) will fire enthusiasm in others, and so will single-minded integrity.

However, it is of little use to be right if you cannot convince other people that you are right. So truth has to be presented effectively in words, with conviction and confidence.

2
Communication

'Communication means the passing of a message from one person to another.'

Wells (1978)

Spoken communication cannot be considered in isolation. We have to look at other forms of communication, we have to examine how and when they are used, to make the most of the spoken word. But first, what do we mean by communication?

A simple definition is this: communication is the successful passing of a message from one person to another. It takes two to communicate. You can't do it alone and it is not a one-way affair. There are three items: message, sender and recipient. Although disparate they are interlinked, so that communication is all of a piece, an indivisible trinity; take one away and there remains only non-communication. Communication is the act of giving and receiving facts, opinions and emotions; the passing of a message is not enough. In this act or process we can identify 12 principles that are inter-related and inter-dependent.

TWELVE PRINCIPLES

Communication depends on relationships
The style, quality, quantity, and complexity of the message will depend not just on the sender and the recipient but on their relationship to each other and to a common past experience. The word 'communication' is allied to that of communion which, apart from its religious connotation, infers a sharing or participation in common, a kind of fellowship. Communication is a two-way process; block one and the result is not communication but a directive. So communication infers agreement of

identity and purpose, something that we have in common, to impart and to receive. Because of this it is important to appeal to the emotions first, to reason later; to get the context right; to make yourself acceptable as the sender because your personality is imprinted on the message. Communication demands effort, thought, time and a willingness to establish a relationship, whether between colleagues or patients, before a message is sent.

Drucker's (1975) statement that 'we cannot perceive unless we conceive' has more than a grain of truth. No fanatic is convinced by rational arguments; nor is the patient who is biased against modern medicine. So the first question to ask is: 'Can the patient receive what I wish to tell him; is he emotionally able to understand me?' Few people realise the importance of this fundamental question. Yet it is central to the argument of communication. If we agree that communication is the mutual exchange of thought between people, there is the need to have minds in tune.

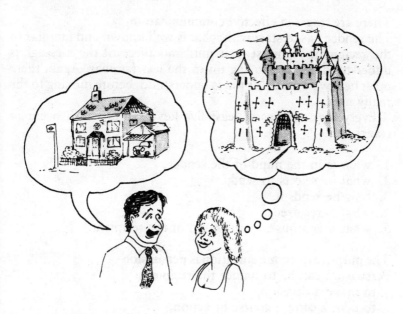

16　*Talking with Patients*

Communication requires certain preliminaries

Before attempting to communicate, the sender will have to think first about the following.

1. Is there a need to communicate?
2. Who is the message for?
3. What is the main aim or objective?
4. How much content has to be included?
5. What is the most appropriate form?
6. How will the message begin?
7. How will the end of the message be indicated? Commonly in speech to indicate the end we ask a question; in writing we use a full stop.
8. What will be the sequence if more than one message is to be transmitted?
9. Is the recipient able to receive? He must be awake, ready and prepared. Hence the timing must be right.
10. Is there enough time to send a complete message? Communication requires time from the sender and the receiver.

There are stages in effective communication

The sender has to start with what is well known and familiar to the recipient. He must wait until this piece of the message is understood before moving on to the less familiar. Again there must be a wait until this too is understood, before moving to the really new.

Every message has at least five key aspects which occur in stages:

1. what is in the mind of the sender,
2. what he selects to send,
3. how he sends it,
4. what is received,
5. what this arouses in the mind of the recipient.

The purpose of communication is persuasion

Persuasion can be to induce the recipient:
　　to make a decision,
　　to take a certain course of action,
　　to accept more information,
　　to accept a concept.

Communication 17

Communication is not simply the transfer of information from one person to another, whether or not it elicits confidence, because the information transferred must persuade; if it does not then it cannot logically be called communication. Communication is a means whereby behaviour is modified and a change is effected in an individual, or a group of people, so that the information is made productive and goals are achieved. That is the essence of persuasion. Fletcher (1973) stated that if communication is to change behaviour, the required change in the recipient must be seen by him to have more advantages than drawbacks; otherwise it will not be made, or if it is made the effect will not persist. New information resulting in a change of attitude is usually a necessary prelude to a change in behaviour. Communication always makes the demand on the recipient to take action and if he does not communication has failed.

Yet communication and information are not the same: they are interdependent and different. To a large extent information is based on logic, communication on perception. Information can be useful or useless to the individual; it can be stored and retrieved. Information is usually specific and precise whereas communication is a pattern of relationships, even though useful information presupposes communication. A glut of information may preclude communication even though communication works better the more levels of meaning it has; for instance a fine painting communicates to the viewer at literal, metaphorical, allegorical and symbolic levels. A certain ambiguity and a multiplicity of levels of meaning helps communication, but too many may completely wreck the value of the information.

More and better information does not solve the problem of how to communicate well. On the contrary, too much information stops effective communication. The repetitive and piecemeal communication is likely to be more successful than the single, short, overloaded message even though short sentences with familiar words and active verbs make communication interesting and persuasive.

The message must be in a suitable form for the recipient
There is a choice of form but:

 writing requires a reader,
 speaking requires a listener,

18 Talking with Patients

illustration requires a viewer,
gesture needs to be seen and interpreted,
inference needs experience and judgement.

Some messages are best said, some written, some both written and spoken, but the sender must use the language of the recipient. The written message must be a delight to read. The writing should be lean and clean; points made without excess verbiage; written with the thrift of a miser yet without a telegraphic style, for it has to be understood instantly and correctly by the recipient. Much the same applies to the spoken message.

There is also another form of communication, inference, which we should consider now. It is one of the commonest methods of communication for the recipient, yet probably the most misinterpreted, misunderstood, and can be the most evil form. 'Had a good night's sleep' implies that the previous night was rotten. 'Bowels now normal' carries no information of itself, except the inference that previously they were not but we don't know if this was true.

2.1 Visual communication

1. Often the most creative form of communication and the most compressed. It can provide 'hidden' or unexpected information.

2. Information can be identified quickly; there can be total comprehension.

3. May be entirely diagrammatic: such as travel maps, location maps, temperature charts, symbols.

4. Message can be simplified to bare essentials.

5. 'One picture is worth a thousand words.'

6. Permanent record, easily transported, may not need language.

7. The visual message may be open to more than one interpretation.

8. May give false expectations such as photography of 'before' and 'after'.

9. Often the best remembered communication: a lasting impression.

10. Can replace spoken or written language.

Inference or implication is a perfectly valid means of communication, but it does lay the burden of preventing ambiguity firmly on the speaker.

The message has to be received and understood

To make sure a communication has succeeded, information about its effects, both immediate and subsequent, is needed and in a form that can be analysed correctly by the sender. So how do we know? By the action taken by the receiver. Effective communication occurs when the action of the other person is appropriate and expected. If the

---

2.2 Spoken communication

1. The most effective and the most personal form of communication.

2. Has directness and immediacy, but no permanence.

3. Uses feedback all the time and so words can be repeated, altered, added, or explained as required.

4. Understanding depends on the rate and rhythm of speaking, recognisable pronunciation, clarity of enunciation, suitable choice of words, hearing the sounds and interpreting them correctly.

5. Grammar and syntax must be simple. Short words and active verbs carry more impact.

6. Uses a limited vocabulary, but word meanings can be changed by colloquial use. There is no need for economy of words because speaking is fast but not very precise.

7. Pauses, gesture, changes of rate, rhythm and volume are used for emphasis, punctuation and interest.

8. Logical progression from simple to complex is not necessary: can dodge about with ideas.

9. Sentences need not be completed: they can be finished by gesture or words supplied by the listener.

10. But spoken words are easily forgotten, misquoted or misunderstood.

---

20 Talking with Patients

message is not received or not understood there is no communication, irrespective of its content or the intention of the sender.

The means whereby we discover if the other has received our message is called feedback; the quantity, quality and speed of feedback depends on the method of transmission. In talking we look at the listener to see if he understands wheat we are saying, we watch his changing expression, posture, gestures, listen to his verbal and non-verbal interjections; this continuous monitoring tells us when to stop, slow down, speed up, or repeat what we have said. Perception is the key and depends on four factors:

the nature of the stimulus and its power,
its background or setting,
previous and related experiences,
personal attitudes, feelings, drives and goals.

Ordinarily we are not aware of the process of perception; we do not stop to analyse the incoming sensations or the basis of our interpretation. We see and hear, and then respond in a certain way according to the context. To some extent we see what we expect to see because perception is largely a process of inference based on past experience.

Perception is not a matter of logic; it is experience. That simple statement is of great importance for the patient because he does not and cannot perceive a single specific event: he perceives a pattern, a picture of the whole. A single word to a patient, 'Better?', depending on the tone of voice, the gesture (such as a raised eyebrow and the beginning of a smile), the environment and events of the previous day, may mean, in effect, any one of these:

'You are better, as I predicted, so acknowledge the fact.'
'You are better, even though you did not believe me when I explained all to you yesterday.'
'Are you better, because I said you would be?'
'Are you better in spite of your previous gloom?'
'In truth, are you really better or are we both trying to kid ourselves about your progress?'

2.3 Communication by gesture

1. Speedy: gesture can say more, more quickly, and often more eloquently than words.

2. It can convey emotion and attitudes better than words.

3. Symbolic gestures and mimicry do not need language: the actions to drink, eat, smoke, kiss, wave farewell are easily understood.

4. Can be used at a distance: the wave of recognition.

5. Reinforces and colours spoken words for emphasis, sincerity and confidence in what is said.

6. A smile and handshake establish rapport easily and do not require language. A touch that comforts requires no words.

7. Feedback occurs and may be by a complementary gesture or speech.

8. Gestures are fleeting and so can be missed or misunderstood.

9. May convey hidden feelings or reveal more than desirable.

10. Avoid professional acting: never be a 'ham'.

Without these added non-verbal gestures, the single word 'Better?' has virtually no meaning and does not communicate. The way it is said, with warmth or coolness, conveys the message. An old adage states: 'No-one can communicate a single word: the whole man comes with it'.

No-one can perceive what he is incapable of perceiving. The reverse is more to the point: we only perceive that which we are able to observe and understand. So we have to learn, consciously or unconsciously, to talk with patients in terms of their own experience, for we can only communicate with another in the recipient's own language and in his terms.

The message has to be clear, simple and unambiguous
Many things in medicine are the exact opposite of this. Yet we have to simplify and clarify if we are to transmit ideas, information, attitudes and emotions from one person to another.

22 Talking with Patients

To be effective, we have to use:

short sentences,
simple words that carry our thoughts with conviction and
 clarity,
short words rather than long, which take less time to read,
 less time to hear and less effort to understand,
illustrations, by pictures or gesture, to clarify ideas as they
 unfold.

Communication must be matched to the knowledge, social background, interest, purposes, and needs of the recipient. It requires empathy, which is 'putting yourself in the other person's shoes'. Communication is effected not only by words, which must have the same meaning for giver and receiver, but also by attitudes, expressions, and gestures. This is especially relevant to a consultation where patient and doctor are both givers and receivers.

Advice on the correct choice of words is often given to those who wish to write well, and we should accept that same advice in speaking. The Fowlers (1962) give five admonitions. Prefer

the familiar word to the far-fetched,
the concrete word to the abstract,
the single word to the circumlocution,
the short word to the long,
the Saxon word to the Romance.

Such advice can be taken too seriously. No two English words express a speaker's meaning equally well and so we have to choose the word which our hearer is likely to understand yet avoid those vague words (such as situation, position, state of affairs) which carry no explicit meaning. When trying to decide whether to make a distinction between words of similar meaning we have to ask ourselves two questions:

Is the distinction worth making?
When the distinction is made will the hearer be expected to
 understand and remember it any better?

Communication 23

2.4 Written communication

1. The slowest form of communication, but the most accurate.

2. Has permanence, but no feedback: essential for drug instructions or advice, medical data reports, appointments.

3. Can be read at will, reread, shown to others, discussed, and the text kept as a reminder or as a warning.

4. Grammar and syntax are formal and the text is structured for the recipient, as in a report, letter, instruction sheet or questionnaire.

5. Uses an extensive vocabulary. Economy of words and their precise meaning are important: too many spoil the message.

6. Logical progression from one thought to another, from the simple to the complex, is the usual composition.

7. Usually an impersonal form of communication and may be interpreted as cold, insincere or unfeeling.

8. Can be transported or transmitted over great distances without alteration.

9. A completed sentence is the unit of thought.

10. It may be produced as evidence in a court of law.

The information must be correct, concise, complete, and in context
Simplicity and brevity are helpful aids for effective communication, but above all the information must have value. The six precepts are:

Convey facts and opinions separately; to mix is to confuse.
Do not convey information already known.
Do not convey information that is not needed at the time for understanding.
Tell all that is needed to understand the message; the amount of detail will vary for each message and each occasion.
Convey messages in a logical sequence.
Do not fling information at the recipient out of context, or out of the blue, because it will be assessed as irrelevant.

24 Talking with Patients

The recipient must be expecting the message

People hear, see and read what they want to receive. They are prepared to receive the expected message, not the unexpected; they will receive the familiar message but may not receive a new message.

Common advice is this: wake him up, look him over, warm him up, then communicate. It is necessary to grab the attention, interest and will of the receiver so that he is switched on, tuned in, and listening. Even then there are difficulties. Think of the enormous gap between different recipients. After a cocktail party, for instance, a husband and wife talk over what they saw. The husband may list the drinks, the food, people he knew and their behaviour. The wife may comment on other womens' dresses, their jewellery, and the room decor. What both have seen was the same; what they noticed was different. They had different expectations, different interests, and different selective memories.

What we can see is based largely on previous experience, and hence the unexpected may not be received at all; it may be seen and heard, but it is ignored, misunderstood or misinterpreted. The human mind tries to fit stimuli and impressions into a frame of expectations. Hence in dealing with patients we must have some idea of the recipients' expectations.

The recipient decides the effectiveness of the communication

He is the final arbiter. The value of a communication is judged not by its purpose or content, but by its effect on the recipient. An elegant or witty spoken communication may satisfy the sender, but leave the receiver uninformed and unmoved. All too often utterances travel to the recipient as a one way system, yet communication can only occur in both directions. It is the recipient who communicates because the so-called communicator, the one who utters, does not communicate unless there is someone who hears and understands.

Utterances travel downwards from doctor and nurse to the patient, but communication travels upwards. The most junior person in hospital must be allowed to pass his information and his opinions to the top executive and not just be a receiver of messages. The success of any message depends largely on the belief already held by the receiver, and the personal credibility of the sender in the opinion of the receiver.

Listening is important but it demands a receptive mind on

the part of the listener, and interjection of questions, so that what the speaker says is clearly understood and interpreted correctly.

The speed of communication depends on the form and mode of passing the message

We can speak quicker than we can write: speech takes place at 100 to 300 words a minute compared with about 30 for writing. Similarly we hear quicker than we can read: we can hear at perhaps 400 words a minute but read at about 80 words a minute. Also, we can see quicker than we can be told: a picture can be taken in and analysed in seconds, speech takes minutes, often for less information.

Speed also depends on the quality and complexity of the mode: clear, concise, simple speech will be understood quickly, muttering long words will not. As Fletcher comments: good communication is brief and to the point, evoking a rapid response. Speed is everything; yet a good message allows only one interpretation.

Communication suffers from interference

Sending a message is not necessarily communication, nor is it enough to think. Admittedly the sender wishes to transmit his thoughts to another but before he can do so he has to clarify them to himself and then encode them suitably for the other. Failure to do so results in semantic 'noise' and incorrect interpretation. 'Noise' in information theory is defined as any factor within or outside a system of communication that alters the intended message (the thoughts the speaker or writer wishes to convey). All person-to-person communication systems suffer interference from noise, but none so much as speaking and writing in medicine.

Writing suffers because the English language is rather ir-rational, and the writer and reader have no channel or feedback between them. The writer must therefore choose his words with care so they convey what he means to an unknown audience whose level of literacy and interest is also largely unknown. The reader may only scan what is written or may read word-by-word to pick up the sense of the message; the former may miss important detail, the latter may be overcome by too much. Medical instruction sheets have therefore to be couched in such

26   *Talking with Patients*

2.5 Non-verbal and non-vocal communication

1. A large collection of um, ah, ers, tongue clicks, breathy sounds, whistles and grunts.

2. Used extensively in conversation; indicates to another it is his turn to speak.

3. Expresses emotions and attitudes of the listener to what is being said with the minimum of interruption to the speaker.

4. Calls attention to oneself when speech is inappropriate or inconvenient.

5. Used for mimicry to give realism to statements.

6. Indicates the listener understands, or is absorbed in thought.

7. A form of recognition of another, often accompanied by a smile.

8. To indicate musical rhythm, or to reinforce a gesture.

9. A generally used signal to terminate a conversation.

10. Regretably, sometimes just a meaningless irritating habit.

a way that they will provide correct information for both groups. Many written documents do neither.

Speech suffers from interferences because we do not use the right word at the right time and we commonly misinterpret the feedback from the listener. The speaker performs three tasks: he gathers information, encodes it into language symbols, and transmits these symbols as signals (in the form of words, accompanied by changes in pitch, tone and volume of his voice). He uses gestures to clarify or reinforce what he says. Speaking, unlike writing, generally includes too many words, repetition and rephrasing. The listener reverses the process: he receives the signals, decodes them into symbols and interprets these symbols as information which he then evaluates. It is a complex process. If the information was incorrect to start with, there is little wonder that it is misunderstood, misinterpreted, or causes confusion in the mind of the listener.

Two other causes of interference with speech should be noted. The first is physical noise from the environment: the noise of traffic, mechanical drills, and general movement of people and objects. The second is the noise of others in proximity talking at the same time. Both may distract the listener or make him lose a vital word in a sentence with resulting loss of meaning of the whole sentence. If this sentence happens to be a key one in the conversation the result may be hilarious or tragic.

COMMUNICATION AND THE PATIENT

The art of communication in medicine is not easy. We communicate with patients by speech, writing, illustrations, gesture, touch and smell; sometimes singly, sometimes all at the same time. The nurse wearing expensive scent tells the patient as much as the doctor with whisky on his breath. The firmness of a handshake carries meaning as clearly as words, in the same way that a smile radiates confidence and friendliness. Good communication carries its own reward: the trust of a patient.

If you do your job well don't expect popularity or even gratitude. You will, however, gain the respect of your patient and as Sir Robert Mark said about the police, it is respect, not popularity, that we want because we sometimes have to make unpopular decisions. If you can communicate clearly and simply the reasons for decisions they are often accepted willingly. If the patient talks to you naturally and confidentally, just like one of the family, then be grateful and proud that you are doing your job well. If the patient is guarded in what he tells you, it could be that you are at fault, by your attitude, demeanour, position or some unfortunate lack of sympathy. Communication in medicine is different from communication in any other field in three important aspects which are seldom mentioned.

Firstly, it deals with an essential aspect of living, called health. Without good health it is impossible to enjoy life to the full. People of all walks of life and all ages have a vested interest (some would say a morbid interest) in any communication that will affect them.

28 Talking with Patients

Secondly, the medical and nursing professions allow the communicator to touch the recipient; not only allow, but encourage such activity. Hence a nurse can communicate readily with a patient in at least three ways: by speech, by gesture and by touch. In all other professions touching the recipient, apart from shaking hands, is disallowed and misinterpreted.

Thirdly, there is a great deal more of a personal and emotional nature in medical communication than in any other. Although confidentiality and trust occur in other professions, such as law and religion, they are of a different nature. The public recognise this difference and those in medicine who reveal the patients' confidential information are rightly censured by society.

'Good communication is difficult. Few can master it without special tuition and constant attention to its effectiveness' (Fletcher, 1973). Effective communication is perhaps the most important attribute of successful medicine and nursing. It is not a secret skill yet it is not always clearly understood nor taught at training school. The principles of good communication are deceptively easy to state, but desperately hard to follow. Here are ten precepts for perfection.

● Be clear in your own mind what you want to put across, how and why.

● Make yourself agreeable to the patient and put the message in the most acceptable form. Early on try to find out if your message means to the patient what you think it means. This is not easy. Probing questions are in order and are necessary.

● Talk the language of your patient and relate your message to his level of intellectual understanding, prejudice, emotion and self-interest. Remember that the patient may not speak your language (not necessarily a foreigner); he may seem to speak your language, but your words may actually mean something else to him. He may have difficulty in listening with attention: from fear, anxiety, physical discomfort, mental confusion, or because of undetected slight deafness.

Communication 29

● Aim to arouse the patient's immediate interest, and then hold it.

● Choose the right medium for your message. If a man is illiterate, it is no use writing to him; if he is deaf, it is no use talking to him. Use as many ways as possible to communicate your message and be prepared to repeat them as often as necessary.

● Choose the right timing, the right intensity and the right length of message, for each occasion.

● Relate your persuasion and your hopes to what is practicable at that moment.

● Use every means to receive and interpret 'feedback' from the patient. Watch his eyes, hands, gestures, and listen to his words, tone of voice, and pauses: each will tell you something. Observe what he does not do, does not say, for these omissions will tell you more. Don't rush. Wait for questions and answer them clearly. Take time, make time, to explain to the patient what he needs to know.

● Remember that communication is a hazardous activity, prone to mistakes, distortion, and misunderstandings. It is a complex process, so always try to simplify what you want to put over.

● Better communication is the key to better nurse-doctor-patient relations; good medicine and good nursing are less important. The difference between strife and serenity often depends on the meaning and on the interpretation of a single word – yours! Successful communication comes when your words are timely, factual, convincing, unambiguous, meaningful and short.

When you speak to a patient, giving a series of well-defined ideas lucidly expressed in words which are right (each idea being linked to the next in a logical order) the message becomes clear, is understood and evokes the response intended. If a thought is clear there is probably one form of words which is best. 'Best' is not an absolute word with defined rules, but

30   Talking with Patients

the most appropriate for the speaker in that context and with that particular patient. The starting point of communication can only be in the mind of the communicator; it can only be effective if the same message reaches the mind of the recipient.

THE SIGNIFICANCE OF GOOD SPOKEN COMMUNICATION

Good communication with a patient is always good medicine. It is therapeutic in its own right, because it humanises treatment and deters ignorance. It provides evidence of professionalism and the right attitude of mind, and can be creative for both giver and receiver. It is the cementing of a personal relationship, and not just a matter of courtesy and politeness. It can be a measurement of mutual trust and confidence, because it is a two-way system unlike TV, radio, or literature, and hence valuable for information, instruction and education that can benefit both the giver and receiver. Good spoken communication is a valuable skill, difficult to obtain because it has to be worked for, and if not practised regularly can be lost. In chronic diseases, or for those patients who require frequent follow-ups, it is essential to establish an easy relationship early on. Good communication carries many advantages, while bad communication carries serious disadvantages for everyone. With good communication it is possible to accomplish more action in the time available.

Morale is good in a team because it creates 'team spirit': everyone knows where he stands, what his duties are and has confidence in his own abilities. Leadership is clear and responsibilities are well-defined. There are less mistakes made than average. The individual, and the team, are more productive than average: more patients are seen, more decisions made, more patients are treated effectively and efficiently. People grow in stature, in their ability and competence. Finally, the hidden potential of individuals is discovered; it is often greater than expected, and can be used in an emergency.

The disadvantages of bad communication are often painfully obvious. Many minor mistakes occur in daily life which quickly become routine, and the risk of grave mistakes increases.

Communication

Morale is low and frustrations are common. It is necessary to repeat quite simple instructions. The output is small because every action carries an element of uncertainty. Delegation of responsibility becomes impossible and inadvisable, because no-one can be trusted.

3
Conversation

'With thee conversing I forget all time
All seasons and their change; all please alike.'

Milton

Few things in life are as enjoyable as a good chat with a friend.
We find that time slips away as we enjoy a good natter. Very
often it is about nothing in particular, and if we are asked later
what we were talking about we have surprisingly little to say
about our conversation. The truth of the matter is that in a
good chat we are not swapping dramatic news all the time.
Indeed, during a relaxed conversation, we are doing a variety of
things – exchanging news, recalling past events, giving our
views, seeking information, spelling out our plans and sometimes just relaxing by talking about anything that comes to
mind.

We lose track of time when we are involved in conversation,
and involved means being interested and playing an active
part. So what is so special about conversation? The dictionary
defines conversation as an 'interchange of thought and
words, a familiar discourse or talk'. It is the informality of the
occasion that appeals to us all, the freedom to start and stop at
will.

Conversation is the opportunity *par excellence* for the nurse
and junior doctor to talk with patients. If the consultant has
seen the patient formally in a clinic he will have had neither the
time nor the opportunity to get to know the patient well, nor
the chance to establish a firm relationship. The consultation, of
necessity, has a formal structure (history-taking, examination
and decision-making) which every nurse and doctor is taught at
training school. Conversation, by contrast, is informal although
it should have a structure which is less obvious; it may be
unscripted, but never structureless.

The consultation or interview is a formal occasion where
straight answers are required from straight questions. Hence the

Conversation 33

gathering of information takes precedence over the pleasantries. In conversation the order is reversed; the occasion is informal or semi-formal at best and the principles and the aims are different.

Good conversation is enjoyable. It also has more serious values: to link people together, to establish or improve human relationships, to achieve relaxation and freedom from worry, to obtain peace of mind which so many patients desire. For all that, few of us prepare or plan what we are going to say to a patient. We have vague intentions. Even in casual conversation you can do some planning; you can think before you speak. Some people are not only unprepared, they actually dread conversation; they are shy when meeting strangers and do their best to avoid conversation. Yet conversation is as natural as sleeping, eating and working. We all need conversation for self-expression, to assert our own individuality, to let others know how we feel, to let off steam; conversation should come easily to everyone.

A monologue is not conversation, but a lecture. Conversation, at its best, means the pooling of information, sharing interests, bringing together ideas. It is a two-way process of give and take, action and reaction. Yet how many doctors and nurses realise these simple facts of dialogue to give the patient a chance to speak? There are ten principles of conversation to consider.

3.1 You and the patient will have

1. Different aims.

2. An accent.

3. Peculiarities of pronunciation.

4. Different vocabularies.

5. Irritating habits of vocal noises.

6. Different sense of humour.

SO BE TOLERANT

34   *Talking with Patients*

TEN PRINCIPLES

● Both parties have an equal chance to speak. Each will have his fair share of listening and talking; if not, the result is a monologue. Bierce defined a bore as 'a person who talks when you wish him to listen'.

● The language used must be understood by both speakers, and will be adjusted for the social class and level of education of the other. Conversation is not possible if the language is not understood and so it is impossible to converse with another through an interpreter. The speaker will use apt words, the telling phrase, vernacular and jargon to make a point only if the other speaker is familiar with these and capable of appreciating their value.

● Signals are used throughout. These may be verbal, or they may be gestures, and pauses so that each knows when to speak and when to listen. You have to talk when it is your turn; if you do not the conversation lags. There is a continuous monitoring of the other, a kind of feedback, which tells the speaker that the listener has understood his words, and tells the speaker when the listener wishes to speak. The rhythm of speaking (you–me–you–me–me–me–you–you–me) is dictated by the subject being discussed and the interest of both parties.

● There is an exchange of information, partly fact, partly opinion, partly fiction. The conversation may start out at a superficial level (the English always talk about the weather, football in winter and cricket in summer) but becomes more serious and more personal as time passes.

● The structure and control of the direction of conversation can be dictated by either speaker, a kind of changing leadership.

● Conversation often includes some reference to the personal interests of the listener (job, hobbies, sport, music, reading) as it becomes more wide-ranging. This is to allow conversation to change course, if either speaker desires.

● Conversation is a voyage of discovery for both parties. Each wants to find out what makes the other 'tick'. Patients will often ask questions which they might not normally (on diet, alcohol, travel and many others) partly for personal information and advice, but more often to discover the attitudes of nurses and doctors.

● Because it is informal, conversation may quite naturally follow the formal consultation or interview (of history, examination, laboratory tests) and become its extension. It is commonly used by both sides to fill in any gap in understanding that remained after the consultation.

● Conversation is a method for developing self-confidence. The effort to talk informally and to listen to the other has been made, and leaves both parties with a sense of achievement.

● Finally, and perhaps the most important, conversation establishes rapport between two people which may lead to mutual trust and harmony of ideas.

It is difficult to write down conversation accurately and truthfully, because gesture alters the meaning of words or replaces them. Sentences are commonly unfinished because the sense is understood and there is no need for completion; sentences may be left hanging in the air full of implications but not words; or sentences may be started in error and corrected by the other person speaking. In novels there is an accepted convention which allows the reader to believe in the written conversation, but the reality is otherwise. Indeed, if a tape recorded conversation is written out and read later it will be impossible to follow or understand, although it was quite clear when spoken.

TEN AIMS

For nurses and doctors, conversation has ten special values, because you can:

● Establish a relationship with the patient. You will have to disclose something of yourself (interests, hobbies, ambitions), to disclose the private you in contrast to the professional you. In a hospital ward, patients will frequently ask a nurse returning to duty: 'How did you spend your off-duty yesterday?' simply because of the personal relationship of belonging to a community.

36 *Talking with Patients*

● Impart information which may be general or specific. It is possible to explain to a patient what his diagnosis really means, to give details of investigative tests (and the results), to provide instruction by inserting a mini-lecture into the conversation, to assert that the patient is in good hands and in the right place and that he will recover from his illness. It is a fact that doctors and nurses are more effective in getting over the message of preventive medicine (that smoking and drinking alcohol to excess cause disease) than all the public advertising.

● Discover information by probing questions, gently of course. On the whole doctors and nurses do not ask enough questions of their patients nor the important ones. How much does the patient know of his condition? Does he understand? What does he expect? What are his worries (domestic, personal, social, occupational) and how serious are they? It is always advisable to talk to a patient about his family and friends if only to discover their attitude to his disease.

● Disclose your own limitations either personal, because you are inexperienced, or general, because there are areas in medicine where knowledge is lacking. It is also fair and timely to describe your own abilities, your confidence in the organisation, your standards of conduct and pride in the professionalism of your job.

● Convey affection and interest in the patient, and get across the meaning of two four-letter words: love and work. The basis of Christianity is two commands: love God as hard as you possibly can, and love your neighbour as much as you love yourself. The Thesaurus lists a dozen alternatives for the word love, but what the patient needs is affection, friendship, charity, the message that you will stand by him whatever happens. And work? Show that every reasonable demand or requirement will be met in full.

● Disclose something of your own personality so that patients will understand better how they stand with you.

● Put disease and hospital in perspective and provide reassurance for the person who finds himself confused by his illness amid strange surroundings. There is a widely held belief, among doctors and nurses, that patients only want to talk about

Conversation 37

themselves and their illness. In my experience this is not true. The majority of patients wish to converse about other things, to establish a relationship and general interest between themselves and their medical attendants, to be acknowledged as people who have diverse interests and skills in the world at large. Admittedly when a patient enters hospital he divests himself of the outside world – his clothes are taken away, he is expected to conform to a new and strange routine and discipline, he is fed, washed and medicated by others, and has little control over how he can spend his day.

To pick up the patient's book from the bed and say that you have read several books by the same author does as much good as asking how the patient feels. To discuss a current topic in the newspaper he is reading, just briefly, will let him know that you and he share the same world, the same worries.

● Listen for clues and contradictions in what the patient says. This may be important and the art of serendipity is discovering the unexpected.

● Have the chance to say thank you, to praise or to chide, to compliment or contradict. Everyone likes to be congratulated (on their appearance, dress, fortitude and so on) and conversation provides the ideal chance to praise the patient for being cooperative in treatment, for accepting a necessary but unpleasant investigation, for putting up with disability or an uncomfortable illness. General Patton once remarked 'All men need a pat on the back once in a while; some need it high and some need it low'. So give praise when deserved and correction when necessary.

One would have thought it easy to say thank you when someone has done you a service, yet most people find it difficult. The service may be as trivial as holding a door open for you to pass, or as great as warning you of professional troubles ahead. No matter. Acknowledgement should be given loud and clear, with a smile and with convincing sincerity. Say thank you so that others around may hear. Never mumble; that's not professional. Better still, if you know the donor's name mention that too ('Thank you, Mr Smith') as a personal appreciation of service; the recipient will know that you mean what you say and be delighted. The sweetest word in any language is hearing

38   *Talking with Patients*

your own name, and it costs so little to say and just a moment of thought. We can all afford that!

● Dispel the loneliness of the patient who has no-one to talk to, no-one to confide in. I always remember meeting a friend who was visiting a hospital where I worked. I asked who was ill. 'No-one', she said, 'I come every week to sit and talk with the patient who has no visitors. We get on fine. He tells me his worries and I tell him mine. I also learn a great deal about the world around me, the kind of information I never knew existed.'

When people fall ill their pride is hurt. They ask: 'Why should this happen to me? What did I do wrong? How will it affect my life?' The questions tumble out and the grumbles too. I was always so fit. I did this and that, yet here I am in hospital! A mixture of crushed pride, unreasonable assumptions, and the sudden realisation that men are mortal. Yet ten minutes conversation can change all that by making the patient welcome and restoring his sense of individuality. The cameraderie in a well-run ward helps too. But the doctor or nurse who converses to bring out the special interest – whether hobbies or work – does far more. Suddenly the patient realises that he is not alone and that it could have happened to anyone.

The good conversation demands a commitment by the patient to the doctor (or nurse) and conversely, because both parties will have to enjoy the encounter, to learn something new and to impart something of importance. They will reach an understanding and forge a special relationship which both value, because they have conveyed their own attitudes to life, to other people and to current events. They have had an equal chance to talk and to listen, and hence to establish their own status. It may be that they have discovered a new world, perhaps only about themselves (that they could converse so easily with an important stranger), and have been stimulated intellectually and found it as invigorating as physical exercise, and will look forward to the next time.

Starting the conversation

When there is a specific purpose to a conversation it should concern one fact alone; the message should be simple, easy to understand, easy to remember, and calculated to arouse interest in the patient. For example, the subject might be how to get well quickly, how to live more comfortably, how to improve in general health, how to adapt to a persistent complaint such as a swollen leg.

What can you talk about to a patient? Almost any topic is suitable for conversation. At the beginning, conversation should be relevant to the patient's illness or condition because a good conversationalist slants his contribution to his listener and stimulates him to talk. So you have to discover the patient's interest which may take time and effort, and you then have to keep the conversation interesting and pleasant which requires a certain amount of steering as you pass from one topic to another.

Be observant for clues which will help you to know your patient. What newspaper does he read? *The Times*, *The Daily Express* or *The Sun*? What books? Look for things you can praise, such as knitting and embroidery or even a jig-saw puzzle, and look for things that suggest a mutual interest. You may have to adjust your own views when talking, but the art of sharing beliefs with warmth and the stimulation of discovering differences requires tolerance.

The good conversationalist finds topics that the patient is interested in. However, before offering a topic for conversation make sure you know something about it. You will not be expected to have an encyclopaedic knowledge about every subject but a good practical one. Week-end golf does not

---

3.2 The five types of short conversation

1. Information: the heart of medical communication and too often a monologue.

2. Social: often little more than a greeting, polite but purposeless.

3. Comfort: often mutual between patients, or between patient and nurse; the aim is clear, to comfort the other.

4. Ritual: an artificial pattern of talk, commonly heard on a ward round and tends to be loaded with jargon.

5. Mood: used to convey emotion between two people. Sometimes light banter or joke-talk is used to cover deep emotions.

---

40 *Talking with Patients*

qualify you to talk about international champions to the patient who is a professional golfer, but you can ask his opinion. You will have to be on the alert for changes in mood and be ready to shift the conversation with them. Notice the patient's facial expression and hand movements. When does he perk up? When does he look vague, uninterested or discomforted?

On the whole shun the argumentative approach, the challenging statement, politics, religion and mothers-in-law. But if the patient wishes to talk about medicine, then let him but do follow the golden rules. The charm of conversation lies in the readiness to pass quickly from one subject to another, not to keep to one topic for several minutes. Lightness of touch is a quality that comes naturally to some speakers; if it does not it is not easy to acquire.

SEVEN GOLDEN RULES IN TALKING MEDICINE

● Speak of what you know. Nobody can know everything in medicine. Hence there is no shame attached to ignorance about the latest treatment of a particular disease, if, and only if, it is outside your own field of work. Better to say you don't know, and will find someone who does, than to fumble your way through inaccurate explanations.

● Talk of what you care about passionately.

● Approach patients through their interests rather than your own. This implies that you learn the patients' interests before you start a relevant conversation. Hence seeking information has to come first. The patient has come because of illness, but is that all there is to it?

3.3 Our three vocabularies

1. Words we use daily and know the meaning of.

2. Words spoken by other people which we understand.

3. Words used for special occasions which we may not understand fully.

Conversation 41

● Don't let the patient wait for information, tell him.

● Start with what is familiar and grasped easily then proceed to the difficult and unfamiliar.

● Tell things, as far as you can, by concrete examples and anecdotes rather than by abstractions.

● Treat you patient with respect.

Put yourself in the place of the patient to realise his difficulties and try to meet them. Never talk needlessly above his head but if you run into patches of incomprehension, back-track quickly and recast or rephrase those sentences; a courtesy you should observe as much in your own interests as in those of the patient. To exhaust every possibility of simplicity is not just good manners but excellent training. On the other hand do not talk down to him; most patients may have more knowledge than given credit for. Above all adapt your style to your patient, so flexibility in approach has to be learned, practised, and remembered.

The patient's limited range of language may be a serious barrier, preventing his access to learning about his illness and its treatment. The doctor and nurse must appreciate this. However, the way into ideas about medicine, the way of making ideas truly one's own, is to be able to think them through and the best way to do this for most people is to talk them through. Hence the importance of conversation between medical staff and patients. Talking is not merely a way of conveying existing ideas to others; it is also the way by which we explore ideas, clarify them and make them our own. In this manner the sum of experience with various patients is built up to become real usable knowledge for doctor and nurse. Talking things over, often quite informally, allows the sorting of ideas and gives rapid practice in the handling of ideas. The nurse who always chats to patients becomes adept at interpreting ideas (of diagnosis, treatment, general management), adept at translating difficult concepts into simple ones, adept at transmitting the essential information in simple and easily understood terms. She is a gem!

42   Talking with Patients

The 'conversational style' of putting across information to a patient should never be under-valued. All too often, the only way to get a patient to think about his illness is to get him to talk about it. Talking is an educational activity in itself. Nurse, doctor, patient – all learn through talking. The first problem is the need to establish an atmosphere in which conversation is possible (a busy clinic with the queue of patients in full view can rarely be conducive to talk) and to build up relationships in which talk is wanted. The casual visit to a ward patient offers opportunity on both sides whereas the retinue of doctor, nurses and eminent visitors on the official ward round does not. We all know, from commonsense and from linguistic research, that genuine talk is not possible in certain atmospheres; nor is it possible in intimidating relationships.

A patient's conversation is most likely to flourish when there is genuine interest in what is being communicated. Fortunately doctoring and nursing are both highly interesting professions to the general public so that snippets of information about previous patients, about research and understanding of disease, opinions on medical TV programmes and on current events do tend to catch and hold the attention of patients. We under-estimate the value of talking with patients about general issues; they have much to learn from us and we have much to learn from them. During such conversations we can create new perceptions, new ideas and new knowledge.

Talk flourishes best when it grows in a context. For the patient the best context is about himself. Talk between patients is largely about their own physical conditions, how they are progressing, an assessment of the accuracy of the doctor's diagnosis and the quality and quantity of nursing that goes with it; sometimes it includes comparisons between different hospitals – but essentially inter-patient talk is self-centred. Many patients are interested in the personalities of those who look after them, however, so they will try to converse on different topics; they may even get annoyed when doctors and nurses misinterpret the situation and deliberately steer the conversation back to the patient's own complaint. Few doctors and nurses seem to realise that the most valuable conversation for the patient may occur when the talk is virtually unstructured, when the ebb and flow of ideas are uncontrolled because 'conversation is the art of getting your own way'.

HUMOUR

A good laugh is one of the few things I can think of that allows you totally to release all self-control and not harm others. Good humour, laughter and cheerfulness are infectious. 'Laugh and the world laughs with you' is an old adage with more than a grain of truth. Curt Goetz wrote: 'Humour cannot be learnt. Besides wit and keenness of mind, it presupposes a large measure of goodness of heart, of patience, of tolerance and of human kindness'. A fair description which points out to the doctor and nurse that humour should have a special place in talking with patients. Carlyle emphasised the humanity of humour when he wrote that true humour springs more from the heart than the head: 'its essence is love; it issues not in laughter but in smiles which lie far deeper'.

Oratory is an art which requires sincerity, skill and enthusiasm. So too with humour, which should have a ring of authenticity about it to be believable. Hence, recounting natural events is often funnier than those contrived. 'Shadow charm' is quickly recognised for what it is because it is not genuine; to overcome this it is advisable to laugh a lot at yourself but not at your own jokes. Never giggle; gigglers are a menace for humour.

3.4 The use of pauses

1. To build up suspense.

2. To isolate an important word in a spoken sentence.

3. For clarity, so that a series of similar sounding words are not misunderstood.

4. To indicate thought.

5. To signal to the listener that he may speak.

6. To allow the listener to catch up with your talking.

7. To indicate uncertainty on how to proceed.

8. As feedback, to discover if the listener has understood.

9. To give balance to speaking, as a form of punctuation.

10. To catch a breath before continuing.

---

44 Talking with Patients

If a patient has told you a good joke, or has a witty description for a particular type of investigation, pass it on and acknowledge the origin. Never make jokes, or clever and disparaging remarks, about staff or other patients because you may easily give offence; in any case it is not professional to do so, nor to make dirty, religious or political jokes.

Never overdo the humour. The patient may begin to wonder if you are capable of taking his illness seriously. Humour is the leaven to the conversation, not the whole. The seriously ill may appreciate a pinch of humour but never a bucketful.

We all use humour, usually for a specific purpose. Jonathan Swift called wit, 'the shortest route to the soul', and that is its commonest purpose. The opposite of humour is not seriousness as many believe, it is humourlessness. Humour is determined by the way we look at people, things, events, and life in general; even if the situation is desperate, there is always a funny side to it. Patients appreciate humour but not a clown; clowns are for circuses, not hospital wards. As with most other things there is a time and place for humour, which has a special value to:

● Reinforce an idea or a point of view, but the humour must be good.

● Relieve a dull or serious situation, or cool an argument.

● Impart a sense of humanity to another person. When we laugh together we become one community.

● Simply amuse and cheer up the sad patient.

● Convey a message, without having to spell it out.

● Decrease pomposity and the importance of an occasion where neither is warranted.

● Dispel alarm, and to dull fears. 'The worst enemy is fear itself.'

● Enliven a conversation which may be lagging, but which should be continued.

● Raise morale.

● Convey friendliness.

Conversation 45

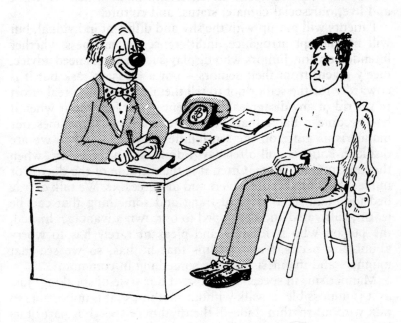

Humour is like a clock. You recognise its value when you see it, but take it apart to discover how it works and all you have is a handful of ordinary words. So humour has context as well as content in conversation.

MANNERISMS

There is a subtle difference between manners and mannerisms. Manners refer to a person's polite behaviour or deportment and his way of handling others. A mannerism is a habitual peculiarity of action or expression which is characteristic of a person. The dictionary implies that mannerisms are signs of affectation. Sometimes they are. But we all have habits of speech, non-vocal noises, and gestures which we use unintentionally; they are part of our personality. In a way they are as distinctive as our finger-prints; they are the outward signs by which one individual differs from another and is so recognised. Mannerisms are the acquired features of our

46 Talking with Patients

character; acquired from the environment in which we work and live, our social climate, status, and culture.

Patients will put up with the shy and diffident individual, but will not accept arrogance, indifference, or rudeness whether intended or not. Juniors who display such features need advice, nicely given, from their seniors – not a pleasant task but it is cowardly for the senior not to tell them. It requires a real effort to get rid of any disagreeable element in our behaviour when it has become a habit that we are unaware of. Sometimes our mannerisms grate on the sensibilities of others and so we are disliked. Patients will often say 'I don't like his manner', when they mean mannerism. Often it is the attitude of the doctor or nurse which has become overt and disagreeable. We talk of 'the bedside manner' as a good thing and something that can be learnt, cultivated and developed to our own advantage. Indeed, the person who is friendly and pleasant rarely has to worry about any peculiar mannerisms that he has, so we see that manners and mannerisms have something in common.

Mannerisms in speech are those of our style of speaking. Just as it is impossible to walk without rhythm, so it is impossible to talk without rhythm. Indeed, the rhythm of speech is part of its expression, and the method of expression depends on the individual. Rhythm is the music of speech, and as such we match it to the emotion to be expressed. Some of us in addition use favoured, colourful words and phrases which express our meaning in an unexpected but interesting way, while others use alliteration and repetition to give a kind of explosive emphasis to a remark ('Don't you dare do that!'). Some speakers use onomatopoeiac words, whose sound imitate or echo the sound being described, such as squelch, thud, clatter. The best speakers have an ear for the right word at the right time, with the gesture which looks right and that's what matters. It is a knack that can be learnt with guidance.

The stamp of our individuality depends too on our phraseology, pronunciation, syllable stress of certain words, and pitch of voice with our changing emotions. Some of these are acquired deliberately, some are developed from necessity, some from the environment at the time, but all have become second nature, a habit, the mark of our style of speaking, our mannerisms in speech. Our mannerisms with gestures, particularly those with the hands, often called gesticulations, depend to a large extent

Conversation 47

on race (the English use less than Italians), sex (females and bangles common), class (the upper crust are more reserved than working class speakers), age (the old use fewer gestures), the occasion (whether happy or sad), and the locality in which we live. They can be distracting to the listener as we talk.

4
The consultation or interview

'Deliberation is the work of many men. Action of one alone.'
de Gaulle

The terms 'consultation' and 'interview' have slightly different meanings, but here they are used interchangeably to refer to a formal occasion.

An interview or consultation differs from ordinary conversation in seven important respects.

● It is a serious conversation with a specific purpose.

● One participant of the conversation tries to motivate the other, to learn facts or to impart information for a purpose.

● An interview looks towards a decision and without a decision the interview may be valueless.

● One participant is always in a superior position. You may argue that in ordinary conversation, between nurse and patient, the nurse is always in a superior position, but this should not be so; the object in normal conversation is to have a dialogue between people of equal status with equal opportunity to speak in turn.

● The interview is initiated by one of the participants, with a specific intention in mind.

● The time and place for the interview are set by the initiator of the interview and there is usually a time limit to the proceedings.

● An interview has much less flexibility than ordinary conversation because the participants must get down to business quickly.

The first consultation is an important medical and social occasion. It should not be hurried. Medical, because this is when the doctor makes the diagnosis, outlines a plan of treatment and the patient can ask a host of questions (and if not, should be encouraged to do so). Social, because this is the time for the doctor to size up the patient and the patient to size up the doctor: the result will be acceptance of each other – reluctant or resolute – or complete disharmony and hopefully recognition that neither trusts the other.

The importance of this occasion cannot be stressed too much. For it is now that the doctor can refuse to accept the other as his patient by tactfully indicating that someone else would do the job better. It is now that the patient can withdraw gracefully and have no conscience of guilt. For all that, the out-patient clinic in a large hospital or the surgery of a crowded general practice are not the ideal places in which to reach momentous conclusions.

THE SKILL OF INTERVIEWING

An interview is a meeting of two people, face to face, to accomplish a known purpose by discussion. If the purpose is removed, what is left is conversation. Hence a conversation with a purpose becomes an interview, which may take place anywhere. A formal interview is one with a set purpose and plan, held by appointment at an agreed place and often with a written record kept; good examples are consultations in out-patient clinics and ward-clerking in hospital. There are four parts to an interview.

● **The aim**, that is the purpose of the interview, can be simple or complex, to do one or more of the following:

to obtain information,
to provide information,
to analyse a situation, solve a problem, specify recommen-
    dations,
to implement treatment,
to remove difficulties or misunderstanding,
to discover the success or failure of a previous interview,
to test attitudes and feelings.

50 *Talking with Patients*

There is a wide choice but the interviewer must be clear in his own mind exactly what he wishes to accomplish.

● **Preparation** is always necessary.

First, be clear in your own mind about the purpose of the interview. Speech should be clear; it should be right, both in meaning and tone. It should also be persuasive. If these qualities are to come through in sound they must be reflected by corresponding qualities in the speaker's mind. Hence prepare before you open your mouth. If you are inwardly unsure of yourself be cautious about speaking; better still, it is wise to say how you feel and that you will have to think about the subject and return later.

If you want to communicate with the patient you will have to obtain information before conveying information. All this means that before passing information there must as far as possible be exact analyses, exact definitions and possible solutions. To handle the patient's problem we must know what it is, state it accurately, work it out correctly and thus arrive at the right answer. If we start in a muddle, or get into one, we cannot arrive at the right answer except by a fluke.

Second, study the subject for interview by having sufficient information or facts before making a start. One may well ask:

What are the main issues to be dealt with?
Should any information be given in advance?
Is it my job or someone else's?
Is the occasion suitable?

Third, anticipate any probable conflicts or special interests.
Fourth, estimate how long the interview will last. Can it be completed within the time available? If not, then you will have to plan time for a further interview.
Fifth, outline a plan for discussion:

Think out the opening statement.
Consider the patient's likely opening question.
Plan intermediate phrases.
Have a written outline if necessary, such as a questionnaire.

Sixth, have everything ready by choosing a suitable place,

The consultation or interview 51

ensuring privacy and eliminating distractions. Give adequate warning of the length of the interview if necessary. Have all documents, data from investigations, x-rays, pen and paper to hand. 'Let me try to find your x-rays' is evidence of poor technique.

● **The structure** of an interview consists of three parts: the greeting; introduction of the subject; and guiding the discussion by question and answer while clarifying and crystallising important points.

The purpose of the greeting is to assure the patient of your interest in his affairs, to show this politely and in a friendly manner, and to put him at ease by reducing tension. Welcome is probably a better word, for that is what it should be; to this end, the interviewer should show a bit of his own personality early on by referring to some item of news, the weather, or something he has done earlier in the day, and thus demonstrate that he is human.

The introduction should indicate the time available for the interview if this is important; clearly one should state the topic in a few words, usually from previous correspondence, and provide essential information so that the dialogue can begin. It is essential to be friendly and confidential, to outline a logical sequence for the interview and to start with a carefully framed question.

Since the object is to draw out information, experience and opinions from the patient, the interviewer must guide and keep the discussion to the subject in hand. It is equally important to encourage the patient to talk, to clear up any misunderstandings on the way and to guide the interview by direct questions and statements. In general, the person who asks the questions controls the interview, but the patient must be given the chance to ask questions and be answered, either as you go along or at the end. The interviewer will, of course, keep an unobtrusive eye on the patient the whole time, for his understanding and responses. It may be useful to summarise each phase of the interview, to establish trust and to clarify the need for further investigations. In general, this stage consists of two parts, obtaining information and providing information.

● **The conclusions** end the interview. Usually the interview is

52   Talking with Patients

terminated by the interviewer who sums up the conversation, states what action is to be taken, checks that the information given to the patient has been understood and indicates whether it is necessary to meet again. Be specially alert during the last few minutes of the interview. The tension should be relaxed, and in an off-guard comment from the patient you may discover significant clues to his personality and his purpose for the consultation. Recognition of both can allow you to conclude with satisfaction all round.

This brief account of an interview, which has many applications, is only the bare bones of what happens daily. Successful interviewing is another matter.

SUCCESSFUL INTERVIEWING

There are roughly seven stages for success.

● Decide on the purpose of the interview. In the out-patient clinic the doctor's intention is to obtain enough information for a diagnosis and then to prescribe treatment. The patient's intent may be identical or quite different, such as to stay off work, to blame others, or to get into hospital. It is naive and unwise to believe that the doctor and patient share a common view, or to deny that patients sometimes deliberately set out to deceive.

● Construct the basic guide to the interview. For the first consultation with the patient, the structure has been laid down by tradition and is well taught at medical schools: history of present complaint, past illnesses, family history, physical examination, provisional diagnosis, special investigations and so on. For an advisory interview (or an explanatory interview with relatives) the structure is not defined; questions have to be put to initiate the required responses that will establish some common ground of understanding.

● Set the stage. This is usually no more than the selection of an appropriate place and the provision of reasonable comfort for interviewer and interviewee. Privacy and quiet are appreciated by both parties but may be impossible in a busy clinic.

The consultation or interview   53

However, when interviewing a patient in a hospital ward it is sensible and thoughtful to conduct business in a side room, outside the ward or in a private office.

● Establish rapport between interviewer and interviewee. On some occasions rapport is established more easily and more quickly than others. You don't have to like the other person, but you do have to deal with him in a civilised and peaceful manner. It is essential that the interviewee feels free to ask questions, not just to provide answers. Indeed, the perceptive interviewer will not just ask for questions but suggest them. The comfortable relationship of rapport can be helped by shaking hands warmly at the start, giving a smile of welcome, and then a few general comments on trivia such as the weather, national news, or some particular local event to ease any tension. It is unintelligent to ask the patient how far he has travelled when his address is in front of you: better to say 'You've come a long way. How did you come? By car?' Then 'How did you manage to park your car here?'

Give implicit or explicit assurance that the consultation is confidential. Always greet the patient by name. If the name is unusual then ask how it is pronounced and where it originated; the response is sometimes very revealing: 'My family originally came from Spain at the time of the Armada' is a remark which cements a relationship (even if you don't believe a word of it) and provides a lead to further questions and a touch of humour on both sides. Start with questions which are the least intimate and the easiest to answer and in this way allay anxiety, suspicion or fear.

● Ask the necessary questions and listen to the response. Efficient technique is important; do make sure that the interviewee understands the questions and finds the attitude of the interviewer acceptable at all times. So, do not look surprised or show disbelief unless these are demanded and useful for further probing questions. It is the interviewer who must make transitions from one subject to another, but sudden changes of direction may be disturbing and erode the previously established rapport.

The patient must see that you are attentive. The interviewer cannot afford to look inattentive because the patient may interpret this as meaning that he has said enough, and will then

54 Talking with Patients

dry up. It is important that the interviewer maintains eye contact with the patient at all times. This does not mean staring at him but it does imply that both should be seated or both standing.

The patient must not feel uneasy when he sees you record the results of the interview because normally in medicine the doctor writes notes as the consultation proceeds. But there are many occasions when such action is inhibiting to the interviewee. There is no 'best approach', but whatever is done should be practical. So, either make brief notes at the time or write a summary as soon as the interview is over. In commercial life the tape-recorder has taken over, but in medicine this seems unlikely if only because of the greater risk of the loss of confidentiality, even though the best record of any interview is a verbatim one.

● Close the interview properly. The way you close matters a great deal; it is important for the interviewee to feel satisfied. So, specific information from the interviewer about future meetings and a strong handshake puts the earlier established rapport on a firm footing. A word of appreciation, or of encouragement, and a light remark all help to close the interview in a friendly manner.

● Interpretation of the interview data. Here there must be caution, because there are sources of bias. The bias of the interviewer is probably the most important because this influences the wording of his questions and his tone of voice. The physical setting and circumstances in which the interview took place may be relevant to the analysis, as well as the emotional state of the respondent at the time. It is all too easy to assess the patient as a fussy, dim, worrier at first consultation, only to realise later that he was a highly intelligent and capable person in unaccustomed surroundings. Do not let your general impression of the patient influence the assessment you have made of him from detailed information. First impressions are often wrong, and sometimes wildly inaccurate. Avoid trying to classify the patient, but try to see him as an individual. Stereotyped patients do not occur in clinical practice, only in novels.

The consultation or interview 55

QUESTIONS

The value of the interview is clearly related to the skill of the one who conducts it; not just the skill of eliciting responses, but the ability to minimise the effects of one's own point of view on the response. There are two types of interview according to the character of the questions.

First, the structured interview where the questions are predetermined and call for simple and direct responses. Taking a medical history is a good example: How old are you? Where is the pain? Have you had any treatment for this before?

Second, the unstructured interview where the questions allow the respondent to voice his opinions, beliefs and attitudes towards his illness: why did you prefer treatment in hospital? How do you manage at work? This form of interview is common in counselling. Frequently the interview will change its form, either during the same meeting, or at subsequent meetings. For instance, the initial consultation in the out-patient department is usually a structured interview, whereas when the patient comes into hospital, and sometimes when seen at follow-up, unstructured questions are used to provide more information to the interviewer.

4.1 Use questions to

1. Encourage the patient to relax.
2. Draw out knowledge, information and opinions.
3. Amplify statements.
4. Keep the discussion relevant.
5. Bring out distinctions and similarities.
6. Reintroduce an overlooked point.
7. Encourage intelligent judgement by the patient.
8. Control the consultation.
9. Discover hidden worries.
10. Check that all is understood.

---

56 Talking with Patients

Experienced doctors and nurses excel by their skill at cross-questioning. So what questions? Certainly, adequate time must be allowed for questions and answers, and time spent listening to the answers saves time in the long run. Questions can be of three types, closed, open, or rhetorical. The rhetorical question does not expect a reply; for instance 'Who cares?' means 'Nobody cares and that's the tragedy'.

Closed questions usually start with who, when, or where, and the answer is expected to be short. For instance, 'Do you have a pain here?' will be answered 'yes' or 'no'. Open-ended questions may start with why, what and how. 'Tell me about the pain' although apparently a command, is in effect an open-ended question which may evoke a long answer. In general, the shorter the question, the longer the answer from the patient, but the length of answer is largely decided by the type of question.

A leading question, not the same as a principal question, is one which is put in a friendly manner and so phrased that the patient is guided to answer in a way which he might not have thought of doing without such help. Patients have to be prompted often and there is nothing disreputable about that. The trouble comes when we weigh the value of a particular answer; it may be necessary to ask another question in a different form to appreciate its worth. In medicine, diagnostic competence depends largely on the ability to follow up a promising lead effectively, and the lead invariably comes from the patient.

Questions are asked commonly for one of four reasons.

1. For explanation of a statement made by the patient, to place events in time, place or sequence.

> 'When was this?'
> 'Where was that?'

2. For more detailed information of the patient's troubles. Often the question is for clarity alone, but may be an exploring or probing question.

> 'Tell me more about your pain.'
> 'I'm not sure that I understand what you mean by ...'

The consultation or interview 57

3. For provocation of the patient, perhaps to make him defend a statement he has made already.

'Really? Don't you think that strange?'
'If you change your job, do you think you will get better?'

4. To express a personal point of view or some contradictory evidence, and for indicating understanding.

'Did you think I would believe that?'
'I see. Then what happened?'

The brief question does not necessarily imply a brief answer, but usually it does infer that you have thought out the question before asking it and chosen your words with care.

LISTENING

Of all skills, listening is the least researched, the least specifically taught, and the most abused. Yet patients expect doctors and nurses to listen to them, if nothing else. And on the whole we don't (Cartwright 1964). However much the practice of medicine changes in the future, listening will still remain important. We do not have the scientific knowledge to measure listening skills, but the patient makes his own judgement with fair accuracy. It has been estimated that students listening to lectures comprehend less than half of their basic matter (Wilkinson, Statta and Dudley 1974), so how does the patient fare when you talk with him? The difficulty of listening is commonly underestimated and few people realise that listening is not a passive act; fewer still realise that in conversation listening is required from both speakers. Indeed, one could say that the art of good conversation lies in the ability to listen with perception.

So here we have two problems: how can we make the patient listen to us, and what do we have to do to learn to listen.

We can make the patient listen by:

● Capturing his attention by discussing what he wants to know.

58   Talking with Patients

● Holding his attention by using simple terms and the personal approach: 'You have bronchitis. You will have to stop smoking'. You, you, you.

● Involving him by making him take some action, such as writing down the diagnosis of his condition. There is an old proverb which says 'I hear and I forget; I see, hear, and do, and I remember'.

● Asking him to analyse what he thinks is wrong with him and then coming to a decision, say about treatment, after discussion.

● Occasionally asking if he has understood what has been said.

● Repeating the essential points you have made.

● As some doctors do, asking patients to repeat the advice they have given them; others such as Fletcher (1980) suggest that details of treatment should be provided before giving the diagnosis.

Listening requires concentrated attention. If you don't understand, ask a question and listen to the answer. Listen again to the patient and look him in the eye. You may now have information. Listen and question, and put yourself in the patient's shoes; do that and you have empathy. Questions should go for quality not quantity, so put the right question and don't presume the answer. Anyway, you will have to analyse the answer, to separate the important from the unimportant, to get at the heart of the matter. In the end you have to find the answer to the question: 'What's wrong with this patient?' That's the nub.

The art of listening
There are two great bars to communication: not taking time to talk to the other, and not listening to what is being said. So the message is simple. Talk and listen, listen and talk, a rhythm for success which goes like this: me, you, you, me. The wise one will make sure that there is always more 'you' than 'me' in the mixture. To entertain some people you only have to listen. Listening is an art. One of the problems of communication arises from the fact that many people do not listen closely to

The consultation or interview 59

what others have to say, but doctors and nurses have to learn to be good listeners as well as good talkers. Here are ten aids.

● Concentrate the mind to listen with complete attention to what is being said.

● Focus your thoughts on the words spoken.

● Listen actively. Passive listening is common, easier, and useless; words pour over you like water over a stone, leaving no impression.

● Show reaction to what is being said, by a nod or a smile. Don't be afraid to show your feelings.

● Do not try to think too far ahead while listening.

● Be alert for the unexpected remark.

● Do not interrupt the other person's speech or be anxious to cut in.

● Listen politely to the patient and give him his say. Conversation means give-and-take, so give the patient a chance by using short and crisp replies when you can.

● Show that you understand, or don't understand, by facial expression and other gestures and the sympathetic grunt. Your own comments can refine what the patient has said, whether this is a statement of fact or the expression of an opinion. Fact and opinion have to be sorted out as you go along.

● Encourage the patient to continue to talk, showing you are following his words carefully, but using link words such as 'go on', 'then what?' Few people are proof against the flattery of rapt attention. Listening to a patient is therapeutic for it may be just as important to the patient to unburden himself, of fears and worries, as to provide the important information about his illness; he will do this during relaxed conversation, so you have to appear relaxed yourself. The first duty we owe to patients is to listen to them. If we do not listen then how can we expect to discover and understand their feelings and knowledge about their illness?

60　*Talking with Patients*

SOME ANSWERS

The answers to patients' questions need not dispel all doubts or go into great detail. The patient who asks 'Is it cancer, doctor?' doesn't always mean it. In my experience (and that of Brewin, 1977) most people prefer not to know they have cancer. They are content to suspect and can then dismiss the possibility later: 'If I have survived all these years since operatiion, it could not have been cancer'. This is not very logical, but comfortable thinking all the same.

Having asked so many questions of the patient, answers to his spoken and unspoken questions should be provided. The patient can only be interrogated for a limited time without becoming tired, so there comes the right moment to provide answers to his questions. No news is not good news for the patient, as Fletcher (1973) and Reynolds (1978) have so clearly pointed out. Giving information is very important. The pertinent information at the first or second consultation should be the material that we so often forget to mention.

What investigations are to be done, why, and what is involved? A few minutes' discussion can make all the difference to the patient's peace of mind.

What did the investigations show and what are the implications? The results should be described one by one. Commonly a chest x-ray is taken before a surgical operation, yet no-one tells the patient what was found. It takes about five seconds to say: 'The x-ray shows that your lungs and heart are normal', a statement which may save the patient much distress, for how can he know that 1000 chest x-rays are taken routinely each year in your hospital with less than a one per cent chance of finding any abnormality?

What is the diagnosis? Use a simple name – if there is no alternative word then write it down for the patient – and a simple explanation. Whether the patient is knowledgeable or not he will have to explain the diagnosis to his work-mates and relatives and it is better that he knows more about it himself than they do. Avoid frightening diagnostic labels at all costs. Oh yes, the patient may say that he wants to know the truth, but truth tempered with mercy is surely good practice. Life is difficult enough already and may so easily become unbearable without hope. Hope is a peculiar thing, a mixture of ignorance,

4.2 The right word

1. Means exactly what we wish to say: it is apt.
2. Its meaning relates to other words in the sentence.
3. Medicine has 5000 special words: write down the unfamiliar term.
4. Short words are better than long: quicker to say, easier to remember, shorter to write.
5. Has no substitute, so repeat it.
6. Is often memorable.
7. Discloses the intellect and originality of the speaker.
8. Is rarely misused or misunderstood.

---

disbelief, expectation, desire, anticipation of the good to come, and the personal reward of having lived an exemplary life. When it comes to giving the patient his diagnosis, tact and a kindly humanity are paramount. It is better to say heart attack than coronary thrombosis; seizure is better than stroke; growth is better than cancer; high blood pressure is better than hypertension; and nervous headaches is better than anxiety neurosis. Not only are the words kinder, they are easier to understand.

What is the treatment to be? Reassurance may suffice but if the patient is prescribed a drug he must be told how often to take it and when, and given some idea of the possible side effects. In some clinics a printed sheet is given to the patient to take home and study – a good idea – but do remember to ask him to bring it to the next consultation so that you can check that he has fully understood the directions. If a surgical operation is required it is kind to indicate when it will be done and briefly to discuss the major possible complications.

What is the outlook? Most people have a greater fear of disablement than death, and of disfigurement too. They will want to know what kind of restrictions on daily life you would advise: job, exercise, habits, alcohol and sexual activity. A patient may mention none of these even though they may be uppermost in his mind; you have to raise the subjects or answer the unasked questions.

62 Talking with Patients

Ask for questions. There should be none if you have judged the situation correctly. But make it clear that if there are any queries the patient can write, telephone, or raise them at the next meeting.

Finally, disposal. State when you wish to see the patient again and, if possible, why. 'I'd like to see you in six months to check on your progress' carries a different connotation from 'I'd like to see you in six months, to keep in touch'. For those with skin cancer, including malignant melanoma, I like to tell the patient that it is in order for him to return at any time if he is concerned, without the need to go through his general practitioner or anyone else: 'Just write or telephone: I'm here every Wednesday afternoon'. The sentence is simple but is an assurance of future help should it be required.

5

Special people, special occasions

*'Because verbal exchanges are man's crowning glory, all other
forms of contact are viewed as somehow inferior and primitive.'*
Morris, Collect, Marsh and O'Shaughnessy (1979)

Physical disability is common in hospital patients. Naturally
there are variations in the degree of incapacity, but there are
groups of patients with disabilities which markedly affect the
way we normally talk with them. They are the deaf, the blind
and the speechless. There are further groups of people who
require a special approach: children, relatives and foreigners. In
addition, we should consider teaching, research, and informed
consent.

THE DEAF

Not everyone with an ear-plug is deaf; one of my patients
listened to pop music throughout a consultation. But about
20% of the population have some deafness and about half of
these are seriously affected. Old people do not like to admit any
hearing loss even when it has become socially embarrassing.
Deafness in patients is usually not immediately obvious and has
to be discovered. If, however, the patient is wearing a hearing
aid be sure that it is switched on and the volume adjusted
correctly. Many older people prefer to switch off at times, either
to conserve the batteries or more likely for some peace and
quiet. A hearing aid does not restore defective hearing to
normal, as many seem to think, because speech is still slightly
distorted. There are seven points to remember when talking to
deaf people.

● Do smile a greeting and face the patient when you speak so
that he can lip read. Even those with normal hearing can hear
and remember more if they can see the speaker's lips. If you

64   *Talking with Patients*

speak with your hand in front of your face or bend your head to write you deprive the listener of more than you realise.

● Speak slowly but not loudly and do not contort your face or exaggerate your lip movements.

● Stop talking when you turn away from the patient or move behind him. But tell the patient what you are going to do before you do it.

● Make sure the patient can see you when you talk and does not have to face a bright light. Make sure that there is no extraneous noise in the room by closing the door or asking others to be quiet. Even normal people lose half of what is said in noisy surroundings.

● Make use of the appropriate facial gesture to reinforce what you say. Keep your hands still so that you do not distract the patient's attention from your lips.

● Talk in simple language. Use short words, short sentences, and pauses between to make sure that the patient understands. If he does not, then repeat the statement or question, or rephrase it.

● Write down all difficult words, appointment dates and prescriptions, and give the patient an instruction sheet for even the most simple forms of treatment. Let him read this while you make a note that he is deaf, and see if he wants to ask any questions. Deaf people can talk.

THE BLIND

Like deafness, blindness can be a relative term. Some people dislike wearing glasses, and put up with foggy vision for the sake of appearances. Hence, if you provide written instructions for patients, watch how they read them. The totally blind, a minority in the population with defective vision, may carry a white stick as a form of identification or come with a friend who will discretely explain. Seven points to remember:

● Blind people can hear. So always talk to the patient directly but not loudly. Never make an indirect remark because blind people can hear better than most; they have to.

● Greet the patient with a hand-shake or touch on the arm, say who you are and mention others around you.

● Always say what you are doing and what you are about to do. Try to keep talking like a radio commentator when you move about and mention objects that you place near the patient.

● Always make sure that there are no steps or equipment in the way when the blind patient has to move, and tell him before you get there.

● If you want the patient to move, for example to a couch, tell him to stand and give him your arm to hold. Do not steer him as you would a motor car. When you reach the couch put his hand on the couch and allow him to get on it in his own way.

● Blind people can speak normally, often entertainingly, so let them speak and ask questions.

● If you give the patient an instruction sheet, read it to him slowly, before handing it to him. Explain how it can be used as a reminder, for others to read.

THE SPEECHLESS

We can use this term to cover those who have lost their speech, say after a stroke, those who can manage a few words because they are dysphasic, and those who can speak reasonably well but with an impediment. Some may have a handicap with expressive speech and some may also have trouble understanding language; it is important to distinguish the two. Remember these seven points.

● Talk more slowly than normally and face the patient so that he can lip read. Do not shout. The patient can hear and understand.

● Do not 'talk down' to the patient, do not treat him as an idiot and do pay attention when he speaks. Do not talk to a relative when you should be talking to the patient.

66   *Talking with Patients*

● Do not try to finish sentences for the patient. Be patient and relaxed. Give him time to find the right word.

● Encourage the patient to write down what he wants to say. You should do the same with important instructions. Get him to write down questions before the next visit.

● Keep questions simple avoiding a choice, so you have to pose two questions for one: 'Do you have pain before meals? Do you have pain after meals?' is better than 'Do you have pain before or after meals?' Go for yes/no answers.

● Do not pretend to understand the patient when you do not. You must understand your patient for otherwise you are wasting your time and his.

● Speaking can be tiring for the patient so give him a break. For some patients a monologue of the plans for treatment is often a good idea.

CHILDREN AND PARENTS

Now that doctors and nurses in training are obliged to attend a paediatric unit, communication with children is practised reasonably well by most. There are seven points to remember.

● Put the child at ease by shaking hands, asking his name, talking about his friends, and asking about his progress at school. He should be made to understand that he is the patient and not his parents, if they are with him. Always talk with children by using their first names. Ask 'What does your mother call you?', 'What does your father call you?' to discover a diminutive or pet name; then ask if you can use it too.

● Always talk directly to a child. Ask him questions which he can answer on his own. Look to a parent for confirmation or reply only when necessary.

● Say what you are going to do before examining the patient. Children put up with discomfort if they know what to expect.

● When explaining the diagnosis or plan of treatment to the parents, include the child in the discussion. Apley (1980)

Special people, special occasions 67

suggests that it is often better for the doctor to turn to a junior colleague and explain everything in simple terms before turning to explain again to the family; this double explanation is remembered well.

● Talk with a child as you would with an adult, and do not disregard information volunteered. Always listen to what parents have to say about their own child; they are good observers with a vested interest in truth.

● Children ask a lot of questions because they are learning about life. Try to answer them truthfully and sensibly.

● The relaxed child talks spontaneously and often.

For children with a fatal illness there is no need to evade the truth. An adult attitude will do because we are all children at heart. There is no need to pretend that we do not fear pain, fear loneliness, fear the meaninglessness of our life when death threatens. Be open, be adult in discussion. There is no proper method of informing a child but parents do have the right to be the first to tell their own children of bad news. If the parents do not, then ask them if they would like you to do so. You will need all forms of communication and much confidence to put the message over kindly and tenderly. You will have to keep talking and listen. You will have to respect a child's confidences and keep his secrets.

Children mature during an illness, and sometimes parents do too. But when an infant dies, it is wise to consult with both parents in case the marriage dies too by default: some parents feel better if they can tell others off or blame another, and it may be better that this happens to medical or nursing staff rather than to the marriage partner. Parents go through the stages of grief (shock, anger, depression, and acceptance) until relief follows and this is not shameful.

TALKING WITH RELATIVES

Doctors and nurses often fail to deal properly with the patient's relatives. It is too easy to assume that all relatives are well-intentioned dutiful people and not bother to ask questions

68   *Talking with Patients*

about their relationship to the patient. Commonly a ward notice limiting two visitors to each patient at a time is thought to be enough protection, without realising that relatives might be a valuable resource in patient management. So here are seven hints.

● If you visit your patient when his relatives are present, introduce yourself by name, smile, shake hands and proudly proclaim your relationship with the patient: 'I'm Dr Sprite, House Physician to Professor Mole who is looking after Mr Smith.' (The patient will look important and pleased.) Most patients will be grateful to you for doing this, and talk appreciatively afterwards, because they feel embarrassed with their folks around and do not know who to introduce or how. The doctor or nurse who makes the first move relaxes the tension, often makes friends, and will be remembered for this kindness.

● Always learn the name and relation of the patient's visitor. You should be prepared to discuss the progress of the patient's illness publicly with his visitor if he so wishes; you will need to speak in general terms but can keep the conversation on a personal level by referring to the patient and his visitor by name as you talk; people are more attentive when they hear their own name. Try to include everyone in the conversation.

● Be prepared to discuss the patient's diagnosis, prognosis and treatment in private with his nearest and dearest relations but make sure of his tacit approval beforehand. In some instances you may have to ask permission ('Would you like me to have a word with your wife when she comes this afternoon?'). On these occasions it is worth assessing the 'value' of the relations for the benefit of the patient's treatment and then enlisting the necessary cooperation by openly discussing what is needed. A relative can play an important part in the patient's recovery and we tend to miss good opportunities.

● Ask relatives, privately, if the patient has any particular worries or is unhappy about himself or his treatment. A patient may well say things to a relative that he would not dream of saying to a nurse or doctor for fear of causing offence or seeming ungrateful. Yet, some of these may be important and easily put right. Ask the relative's advice about social, domestic

Special people, special occasions **69**

or personal problems that might be troubling the patient. Confer and decide how they should be solved.

● Secrecy and confidentiality are not the same. You must not pass on confidential information to a relative unless the patient specifically requests this. But there is no need to be secretive about matters which should be discussed openly such as a fever, slow progress, good progress, likely time of discharge and many others. It is right to praise the good qualities of the patient in front of his relatives, and to compliment them on their good fortune or on their earlier care for the patient. It always pays to point to the good features of the personality of the patient, as it does to point out the hopeful signs in his illness while never omitting to mention privately later to the relatives those features which are worrying and ominous.

● If the patient is aged and obviously dying, he may welcome death, not just as a release from pain but from the tedium of living. Relatives may not appreciate the seriousness of the patient's illness and will have to be told tactfully; they may not understand the patient's attitude and this too needs explanation. Relatives often have a sense of guilt which they will want to talk about, and quite reasonably want to know if 'anything more can be done'. A doctor and nurse who appreciates this attitude will gain a reputation for kindness just by listening.

● When the patient dies, it is the relatives who grieve, who want to talk, who cry to be comforted. Comfort is supplied by talking with them and listening to their lament in a quiet and comfortable room, by offering the hospitality of a cup of tea or coffee, by arranging for them to see the nurse and doctor who looked after the patient in the final hour if that is indicated, by being helpful and informative about travel, accommodation, and the more formal procedures required at the time. Offer to make telephone calls, if only to call a taxi. Think ahead. (See also Chapter 8.)

FOREIGNERS

Medicine is international. Hence some non-English speaking patients are likely to be seen in hospital or general practice and even those who have lived in the UK for 30 years may still have a poor command of English. Joy Parkinson (1971) has provided a book of terminology for overseas doctors and for foreign medical students taking examinations. Anderson and Ward (1979) have produced *English Tests for Doctors* with three tape cassettes. But for dealing with the patient seeking medical help there is no such guide, so here are seven hints.

● Do speak slowly, clearly and not loudly.

● Keep it simple: use active verbs, concrete nouns, few adjectives and adverbs, and short sentences. Avoid medical jargon and idiomatic English. Repeat the same sentence if it is not understood. Remember that it is easier to understand speech if one word is used instead of several, provided the meaning is unchanged by brevity.

● Keep it short. Do not give any unnecessary information and never give too much at one session. Do not condense when a longer explanation would convey information more understandably.

● Use pictures to illustrate what you mean, but do not give examples or comparisons: they are likely to confuse. Use gestures to illustrate speech; these will be mainly mimicry.

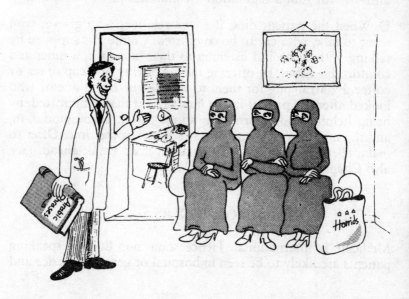

Special people, special occasions 71

● Use many questions but do not use questions where the answer can be 'yes' or 'no', because these may be among the few words that the patient knows (the two other commonest in my experience are 'O.K.' and 'Coca-Cola'). The patient may say yes to please you.

● If an interpreter is used, make sure that he has as good a knowledge of English as of his own language, so talk to him about himself before using his services for accurate translation. The patient must trust the interpreter and his confidentiality. Even then, speak directly to the patient when questioning the patient, but turn to the interpreter when giving explanations. In this way you will learn more about the response by the expression each shows. You will see whether you have been understood, what effects your words have on the other, and whether the advice is accepted. Discuss detail with the interpreter when necessary so that he can translate your message accurately to the patient.

● Be patient. Use frequent pauses for the interpreter to translate easily without having to remember too much. For important statements tell the interpreter to translate each word as you say it. Choose your words to avoid confusing connotations: the word 'sick' can mean 'ill' or 'vomit', so which do you mean? Instant interpretation does not occur at medical consultations, so allow three times as long as usual for this interview.

5.1 Common faults in talking

1. Making things too complex for the listener.

2. Mixing fact and opinion.

3. Using long sentences.

4. Providing too many indigestible facts.

5. Introducing mathematics.

6. Being too brief or too simple.

7. Using long words to impress rather than to inform.

8. Talking impersonally.

9. Speaking too quickly.

72 Talking with Patients

TEACHING WITH PATIENTS

Medicine and nursing are both eminently practical professions. The fact that they are best taught on people and not in the abstract has long been recognised; some hospitals are designated 'teaching hospitals' and more recently postgraduate centres have been built as additions to other hospitals. Most patients do not object to being models but like to be asked permission first; many will have their first experience as a teaching subject in the out-patient clinic.

The routine ward round is part of hospital life: patients come to know what to expect, little preparation is required and it is not much different from having visitors. In grand rounds there may be more detailed discussion on selected patients who must always be warned in advance; they should be told the reason for the extra attention they will receive and for the new faces among the audience. If there is no advance warning, patients may easily become terrified especially when juniors are asked for their views or are questioned in front of them. It is not much fun seeing your 'personal doctor' put on trial and not easy to accept that what he says is right later. It is kinder to warn the patient beforehand not to take much notice of any remarks made because 'grilling' juniors is one way of teaching them and making them think on their feet. It is not malicious, however intense.

The third form of teaching is the demonstration in which an individual patient, separated from the usual ward surroundings and now on his own, is expected to give a stage performance for the benefit of a defined but larger audience at a specified meeting which may be a regular weekly occurrence. At a smaller meeting, a teaching seminar, several patients may be demonstrated in rapid succession, usually to show distinctive physical signs. At larger meetings perhaps only one patient will be interviewed publicly, and even he may make a very short appearance, so short that the patient is left wondering why he has been called. The demonstrator has a key part to play in allaying the patient's natural anxiety, in establishing a friendly atmosphere, and above all in explaining so that everything is clear.

Duties of a demonstrator

The demonstrator has a duty to the audience to present a case in the most interesting and instructive way, to his chief and

Special people, special occasions 73

colleagues to do the job well and with knowledge, and to the patient to act with responsibility and feeling. How is the demonstrator to cope with these three allegiances which may not be identical? His first concern should be for the patient. He should make it clear that everyone in attendance is concerned with the patient's well-being; there is unity of purpose.

● The demonstrator should have obtained the patient's permission beforehand and have explained what to expect and what is required. If the demonstration deviates from the briefing, he should explain to the patient exactly what is taking place; it is bad enough for the patient to have to look at a large audience without having to cope with the unexpected. Indeed, a collection of nameless faces staring at you is enough to make nervous even the most courageous; attending a demonstration is an ordeal for the patient.

● He should not have delayed the patient's treatment, nor over-investigated his condition, nor delayed his discharge from hospital simply for the demonstration.

● He should organise the patient's safe and punctual transportation to the meeting. If the patient comes by car he should have arranged a convenient parking space and have someone familiar to meet him. It is the demonstrator's duty to make sure that the patient returns home or to the ward without delay.

● He must introduce the patient to the audience and the audience to the patient. He should pronounce the patient's name correctly and clearly and use it repeatedly when he is asked questions. If a question is not clear, either because the acoustics are bad or the question is too involved, he should repeat the question to the patient and use familiar terms when necessary. He should translate medical terms to the patient when they are said. When there is an important person in the audience who speaks to him, the demonstrator should tell the patient who it is.

● He must show respect to the patient at all times. A good relationship between the patient and the treatment team is the foundation on which educational demonstrations are built, and this is the only way that they can prosper.

74   *Talking with Patients*

● He must cause no mental anguish to the patient by the use of words which carry serious connotations. He must cause no physical pain to the patient by allowing others to feel a tender area.

● He should make a point of thanking the patient publicly at the end of the demonstration. He should reinforce the gratitude of the audience and of himself privately afterwards, when he should tell the patient of the discussion about his condition and ask the patient for any questions that may have been evoked by the occasion. Although this is no more than good manners, the post-demonstration chat helps to cement a firm relationship. Moreover, if the patient has performed well, perhaps by a witty remark, he should be congratulated. It is surprising how many patients volunteer a repeat performance.

RESEARCH

Research and teaching go together. Lord Moynihan said that every patient presents two questions: What can I do for him? What can I learn from him? Questions are at the heart of research and teaching. The best teaching, and indeed the best clinical care of patients, occurs in institutions with active research programmes, yet the patient must consent to any research done on him.

Much research will be clinical trials of a new drug or a new form of management for his disease. Such trials will need 'controls', that is patients who will receive the currently accepted, appropriate, and the best treatment for their condition; they do not receive 'no treatment'. When a dummy or placebo tablet is used instead of the one being tested this must not be the sole treatment for that patient unless there is no recognised form of treatment for his condition. And there are relatively few diseases in modern times which have not acquired a recognised form of treatment. Whether that treatment is effective is another matter. Others, the 'treated' groups will receive the new medication for which there must be some evidence that it is at least as effective as conventional treatment.

The plan of the clinical trial must be presented to the local ethical committee for approval before any research is undertaken. The application may be approved, but limited to a time

Special people, special occasions 75

or a number of patients, and to one or more responsible persons who will be doing the research. Permission to proceed must be in writing and implies that a report of the findings will later be sent to the ethical committee. There is widespread public disquiet that, while research is recognised as necessary for progress, the ends do not always justify the means. Those involved should be familiar with *The Dictionary of Medical Ethics* edited by Duncan, Dunstan and Welbourn (1981). It has also been suggested that ethical committees do not always do their job (Pappworth, 1978) and that stricter control should be exercised over the methodology (Melmon, Grossman and Morris 1970).

In embarking on research you will need to do ten things.

● Explain to the patient the difference between ethics (a code of conduct) and etiquette (good manners) and then say that your research has the approval of your local ethics committee.

● Describe your proposed research to each patient. Do not ask 'What is the minimum I have to tell this patient to obtain his consent?', but rather 'How much must I say to make the patient understand what it is all about so that he will cooperate willingly with me and be able to explain my research to others?'.

It is often easier to talk to yourself, as it were, in front of the patient and to answer these five questions:

What do I want to do?
Why do I want to do it?
What do I expect to find?
What will it mean for the patient?
What will it mean for other patients?

If you cannot explain your project in simple lay terms you probably have not thought about it enough, and should not be doing it.

● Introduce and specify any collaborators by name. Explain what they will be doing and how they will do it. In some published reports, 50% of the patients did not know who was responsible for the research!

76   *Talking with Patients*

● Obtain the patient's written consent to the research. The consent forms must be held by the chief researcher and be available for inspection. It is unlawful to obtain consent by fraud; self-deceit is morally worse.

● Explain the possible risks to the patient. This does not mean pointing out all the risks that have ever been reported – even aspirin has a bad reputation in this context – but stating the most likely, and say that these will looked for. The gain must outweigh the risk, and the gain must be proportionate to the severity of the patient's disease.

● Indicate that the doctor and nurse in charge of the patient will protect his interests at all times. *Primum non nocere.*

● Tell the patient that he has a right to refuse to enter a clinical trial and will be allowed to withdraw at any time, without detriment. If his progress is unsatisfactory or contrary to expectation the 'new' treatment will be stopped immediately.

● Indicate that detailed records will be kept of all the measurements made, and that the patient will receive many visits. Patients welcome the extra attention and are rarely alarmed by it.

● Tell the patient that he will be kept informed of the progress of the clinical trial and that his relatives also may enquire. It is important to invite and answer questions from the patient and his relatives; there should be no suggestion of secrecy about the research.

● Tell the patient that the records kept will be confidential and that if the results are published he will not be named in the report. It is unwise to even hint of a break-through in management of his disease from your research, rather that a small but worthwhile advance may be made.

CONSENT

Consent is a voluntary agreement to a course of action. Informed consent is required by a patient before an operation, certain invasive investigations, and research; permission (which is a licence to do something) is required from the nearest relative

Special people, special occasions 77

for a post-mortem and for a donor organ such as a kidney, heart or eyes. The agreement is written, contains the signature of the patient or his agent with the signature of another who is usually a doctor, and it is a legal document. The signatures are not usually countersigned by a witness although for certain procedures that may be advisable. Printed consent forms, of a standard design, are usual and continue to be a source of debate among medical defence societies, lawyers and patients. The patients object mostly to the fact that the form does not state what type of anaesthesia will be used and who, specifically, will carry out the procedure; by contrast the procedure is defined, although there may be insufficient space for the inclusion of much detail.

But informed consent? Yes, informed. Impossible. There can be no such thing. If it takes six years for a doctor to qualify and perhaps another ten to reach the level of knowledge of the surgeon who is to carry out a rather complicated operation, how can the patient be so informed in ten minutes? That is the crux. Assisted consent is what is wanted. The patient must be helped to come to the decision to signify his consent; he may have neither sufficient knowledge nor insight. He wants to ask but does not know what questions to ask. He cannot decide values on his own; the nurse and doctor have to help him, but how? Silence does not give consent.

Decision making is planning a course of action with the best available evidence. It is prospective action; it often has to be taken on insufficient evidence and the patient has to accept this fact. In addition, decisions may have to be changed as the quantity and quality of the evidence becomes available. In any case the patient has the right to:

ask for a second opinon on the diagnosis,
refuse treatment altogether,
make a choice of treatment where this is available,
take his own discharge from hospital, or,
seek advice elsewhere.

Aiding the patient to come to a wise decision does not take away these fundamental rights, but helps to extend them and make them more fruitful. The real questions are, how much to tell, who should say it, where and when should it be said.

78   *Talking with Patients*

5.2 Decision making

1. Formulate the problem as accurately as possible by collecting the evidence.

2. Analyse the problem: may need special tests or more questions and answers.

3. Develop possible solutions by weighing the pro's and con's of alternatives.

4. Find the best solution in the circumstances based on the available facts, current knowledge and available resources.

5. Put the decision into practice.

6. Monitor the effect of the decision by checking on the results and consequences of the action taken.

● How much information should you tell the patient?

A certain amount of fine judgement and common sense is needed. Some patients want great detail, others none. If consent is required for a relatively minor and straightforward operation, a simple quick explanation is enough. Use your loaf, be helpful, and put yourself in the patient's place. If the operation is life-saving there is no need to go into every detail but the main risks should be pointed out. If it is not an emergency then the time should be spent talking to the patient so that although he learns of the risks he is not frightened by them. But for research, as described earlier in this chapter, quite a lot of detail is required and often there are special forms of consent.

● When should informed consent be obtained?

Before any procedure requiring such agreement, naturally, but not at the last possible minute. If the patient is seen in a clinic and the date of operation is negotiated at that time, it is sensible to obtain written consent at the same occasion; the patient, often with a relative present, can listen to the explanation, ask questions, talk it over, and even bring a list of further questions when the time for treatment comes. This patient will be well informed. By contrast, the patient who is presented with a paper to sign when already under premedication is likely to be ignorant and unhappy and has reason to complain.

Special people, special occasions 79

● Who should ask for consent?

This job is often left to the most junior person in the team which is a pity. Although there is no need to describe every detail of an operation, every possible complication and every event afterwards in order to 'inform' the patient, it is reasonable to expect information about the most common risks, the most likely complications and how they will be prevented, a little bit about pain or discomfort, and whether there will be any deformity, disfigurement or disability. If this is agreed as reasonable and expected by the patient, then the most junior person is usually not in a positon to explain from personal knowledge. Certainly in research it must be the researcher who asks for consent and no-one else.

● Who should give consent?

The age of consent is that age fixed by law at which a person's consent to certain acts is valid in law. For medical conditions this is 16 years. Consent should always be given by the patient to be treated, unless under age when the signature of a parent will suffice. For research on children parents probably cannot give consent in law, and should not be asked to do so.

Request for consent for a post-mortem on a patient or for donor organs is usually made to the nearest relative, the next-of-kin. This is consent of a different sort, more like permission

---

5.3 **Persuasion depends on**

1. Good communication.
2. Clear advantages.
3. Logical argument.
4. Opinions of other patients.
5. Evidence of benefit.
6. Oratory.
7. Integrity of the speaker.
8. No coercion.
9. Fear of alternatives.
10. Faith.

---

80 *Talking with Patients*

to do something which clearly is not in the interest of the patient. These requests should always be made by a doctor who has played a part in the patient's treatment and so can answer any queries from personal knowledge, and the more senior the person the better. The request should be made in private, and not in the middle of a crowded ward, and only after some explanation of the reasons for the request. It is often an exercise in persuasion, an art that can be learnt but which does require tact and sympathy without an authoritarian attitude. There must never be even the hint of a demand. The success of the persuader depends on two things: the content of the message and how it was put together, and the relative's opinion of the status, prestige, competence and trust-worthiness of the persuader. The latter is important because the message from one person may be more readily believed and accepted than the identical message from another. Some do better than others; they take more time and trouble to talk and go all out to convince the relative that he is doing the right thing.

Finally, never ever persuade a patient to sign consent to any procedure against his will, unless you are certain about two things and have both in writing: that the proposed procedure is life-saving and that an independent second opinion agrees. Patients are just as litigious because doctors and nurses do too much as too little. It is in the nature of things that certainty and a guaranteed result can never be provided. The patient has to accept a certain degree of uncertainty in outcome and this should be clearly understood. But there should be no uncertainty about the intentions of what is planned to be done or about who will do it.

6

Talking about diagnosis and prognosis

'If a man will begin with certainties, he shall end in doubts, but if he will be content to begin with doubts he shall end in certainties.'

Bacon

Butterworths Medical Dictionary defines the word 'diagnosis' in two ways. Firstly, 'the term which denotes the disease from which the person suffers (such as tuberculosis)', and secondly, 'the art of applying scientific methods to the elucidation of the problems presented by a sick patient'. The second definition implies the collection and critical evaluation of all the evidence obtained from various sources and by the use of any methods necessary. The two definitions are complementary. The word 'statistics' is used in much the same way, meaning a system of methods for gathering numerical data and, separately, the actual data.

Even though the desire for cure is uppermost, most patients want to know why they have become ill. They feel that a knowledge of the cause will help the cure. When patients ask 'why?' sometimes they mean 'what is the pathology?', sometimes 'what is the aetiology?' and sometimes 'why should this happen to me?'. The patient may try to provide clues: is it due to worry, strain, a chill, rheumatism, allergy? On the whole is it wrong to accede to any simple but bogus explanation. It is far better to try to describe how a diagnosis is made, to explain that

---

6.1 The three diagnoses

1. The presumptive diagnosis, the most likely based on symptoms, history, physical examination.

2. The working diagnosis, on which management is planned.

3. The definitive diagnosis is an accurate description of the patient's complaint based on all the evidence, including special investigations and treatment.

---

82 Talking with Patients

the evidence has to be fitted together like a jigsaw puzzle. Explain that the jigsaw of disease may be incomplete and require special tests, and that even these may not provide a complete answer. Perhaps, and more importantly, there may not be a single cause but many risk factors. For instance in coronary disease, heredity (a family history will help the patient to understand), high blood pressure, smoking, obesity, and a high blood lipid level will all play a part besides the 'stress at work'.

EXPLAINING THE DIAGNOSIS

We have to explain to patients how the diagnosis of a disease is made. First, from observations: history of symptoms and signs, physical examination, and any special tests. Second, by analysis of the value of the information obtained. Third, by synthesis of this information, to reach a clinical diagnosis which explains all the facts; it is this 'working diagnosis' on which treatment will be based. Fourth, that we may reach a conclusion, the 'definitive diagnosis', perhaps only after treatment has been completed.

All this is based on scientific method, a logical order of observation, followed by a hypothesis to explain the facts. These are then subjected to experimental validation, which may lead to confirmation of the hypothesis or its negation; if the latter occurs we have to formulate a new hypothesis, and re-examine the original observations in a new light. It is a continuous process, and always will be. Even at the end there is no certainty that we have discovered the whole truth.

The diagnosis and how it is made may have to be explained not only to the patient but also to a relative or friend. For instance, in dealing with children it may be necessary to explain first to the parents and later to the child, stressing words of different connotation for each occasion.

The diagnosis may be simple or complicated and therefore require more than one consultation in which to pass on all the information. More importantly, the diagnosis may be of such a serious nature that it threatens the patient's work or life. Under these circumstances it is important to:

● Provide a little information at a time, but as much as can be

Talking about diagnosis and prognosis 83

understood and accepted by the patient. 'Make haste slowly' is a good maxim.

● Recognise that not everyone wants to 'know the worst' even though they may have said so. The patient who indicates that he wants to hear no more should have his wish respected.

● Point out the favourable things at an otherwise gloomy occasion. To the patient with advanced cancer, one can remind him that at least he has no pain and that he has a devoted wife and fine-looking children. For the mother who delivers a child with a cleft lip or palate, I point out that we do make children look good and speak well by modern surgery, and that such children usually have a very nice personality; they are tough physically and psychologically because Nature is kind in compensating for a physical deformity.

● Always provide hope by referring to the patient's present state compared with the past, or by giving anecdotal experiences of other patients.

6.2 What the patient wants to know

1. Is it serious? What is it called?
2. What tests will be needed?
3. When will they be done?
4. What effect will the diagnosis have on my habits, hobbies, social life and occupation?
5. What treatment will be given and what is the outlook?
6. The duration of my disability. Will I be crippled? When can I return to work?
7. What is the significance of my symptoms: what should I look out for?
8. What is the purpose of any pills?
9. How can I help in my recovery?
10. When should I return for a check-up?

---

84   *Talking with Patients*

● Give the patient a chance to ask questions by saying 'Is there anything worrying you?' or 'Is there anything else I can do for you?'

● Interview and make an ally of someone whom the patient trusts and will confide in. Curiously a patient may not discuss his serious illness with his wife (and the reverse is true) even though both are fully aware of the diagnosis and what it means. It requires skill and much diplomacy to make the two converse without fear, but the rewards can be great all round; the patient and his relatives are relieved of unnecessary secrecy, feel happier, and commonly pull together for the patient's benefit.

FIVE USEFUL GUIDES

There are no rules on how best to explain an illness to a patient but here are five useful guides.

● The language barrier: medical terms will have to be turned into everyday words for understanding. Clarity is vital. So, the use of examples and comparisons are helpful even if one word has to be replaced by many. Clarity takes precedence over brevity – so no jargon, ever.

● The patient should have his anxieties dispelled as soon as the correct diagnosis becomes evident. The diagnosis and management should be explained in simple terms often with diagrams which he can retain and study at leisure.

● Repetition of information already given may be a bore, but again it is often necessary. We now know that less than a third of difficult information provided at one consultation is retained by any patient; hence repetition is understandably important.

● One doctor only should explain the diagnosis to the patient, not a group, so that the patient will not be given conflicting information.

● Always give the patient the chance to speak to you alone; the doctor must never appear too busy to listen or to talk. Many patients lack the courage to ask, some do not know how to ask, and some really do not want to know. The inaccessibility of a consultant on a ward round, surrounded by others, invokes

Talking about diagnosis and prognosis 85

frequent and adverse comment by patients, particularly after they leave hospital. It is very reasonable to nip round the wards on your own afterwards, unaccompanied, so that those patients who need a word or two will have the chance to utter them, a practice I strongly recommend. Of course, one has to be selective and decide who really needs to be seen again.

WHY MUST THE PATIENT KNOW THE DIAGNOSIS?

Every patient should be provided with a label for his condition, the correct diagnosis, because firstly it serves as a respectable explanation to others to satisfy curiosity of what is wrong, to explain why the patient cannot work, why he is not his usual self and not taking part in his usual activities. Second, the patient needs an explanation for himself that accounts for his personal feelings and the condition of his body, and to give him some insight into his disease. Third, the diagnosis is a method of retaining self-respect when ill, and a personal comfort, because knowing the diagnosis helps to make the illness more tolerable than a nameless fear. Fourth, it serves as an assurance that doctors and nurses know what is wrong and how it can be cured. It gives the patient the chance to acquire information from friends or even total strangers about his condition now that it has a recognisable name. Fifth, it acts as a warning, because sometimes ignorance can be dangerous, and so it is a pointer to true north: the correct and timely diagnosis should lead to the selection of medicine, physiotherapy or surgery that is likely to be helpful and may restore the patient to normal living. Sixth, the diagnosis is a label of convenience for patient, nurse and doctor when conversing; a name to bandy about, but its meaning must be understood. Finally, it prevents the patient acquiring a false diagnosis. As G.K. Chesterton once remarked: 'When people do not believe in God they do not believe in nothing; they believe in everything.' So too in medicine.

CONSEQUENCES OF A DIAGNOSIS

In other words, what follows a diagnosis? There may be three different events.

86 Talking with Patients

● Treatment, and that is dealt with in the next chapter.

● Further investigations, to prove, disprove, confirm, or refute a presumptive diagnosis and to provide enough information for planning treatment. The investigations should be named and written in the case records in front of the patient. The patient should be told what each separate investigation involves and what it is for; difficult terms should be written down for him. And when the results come back he should be told in lay terms what each test showed and what it means; failure to do so may make the patient suspicious that the test has disclosed something so dreadful that it could not be passed on. It is better to use the term 'normal' for those results which are recorded in numerals within an acceptable range. To quote an exact figure for, say, a haemoglobin of 14.4 can worry the patient who was given the figure 13.1 a month ago. Indeed if the patient insists on knowing the figure the informant has a duty to discuss the ranges of normal and the errors of sampling. Quite a task.

● A second opinion, either for making or confirming a diagnosis, or for general management. This action will require some explanation to the patient. Firstly, why the doctor wants it ('Your condition is a little outside my field, but Dr X has made a special study of it and really is the expert in this country/ locality'). Secondly, why the patient should accept it ('Dr X will be able to give you better advice than I because of his special interest in your condition').

If specialism means anything, it means the individual patient shall benefit from the best expert and not from the second best. Not everyone will agree. The practical result of multiple second opinions is that the patient can become confused by the number and variety of doctors who come to see and examine him. Who is in charge? Who will answer his questions? Who is the leader, the top man to whom he can refer for advice? Regrettably, in modern medicine, the answer is no-one. It is no wonder that patients who receive marvellous treatment express dissatisfaction and complain that they have not been told. The modern habit of passing a patient from one doctor to another, without making it abundantly clear who is in charge, is to be deprecated. This is bad manners, bad medicine, and in the end often bad

Talking about diagnosis and prognosis 87

treatment and bad management of an ill and confused patient who has been passed on like a chain-letter.

The lesson is simple. The doctor and nurse by whom the patient is first seen shall remain in charge until there is a clear transfer of authority for treatment and this is explained in detail to the patient and understood by him; and, as an act of friendship, a subsequent visit is made so that the transfer is seen to be satisfactory on both sides.

PROGNOSIS

If a full explanation has been given at the time of diagnosis and a further explanation of the necessary treatment, the need for extra information on prognosis is narrowed down to about three questions. But the answers to these are haunted by five other questions which the doctor and nurse must be able to answer to themselves.

How much does the patient already know?
Has he understood what he has already been told?
How much does he want to know?
What must he be told?
What is he afraid of?

Without a fairly clear idea of the answers to these five questions, depending as they do on judgement and knowledge of the patient and his disease, it is difficult to discuss prognosis sensibly. The answers to the first three questions are commonly revealed in conversation, by gentle probing; the answer to the fourth should be clear from the diagnosis of his condition, but the answer to the last may require some clever detective work.

Most patients are prepared to pay a lot for peace of mind. They will accept the revelation of a fatal illness, and thank you for telling them, if put gently and kindly. Here, previous personal experience counts. But you must negotiate the price before you speak, and that too is discovered in conversation. Prognosis should be considered as part of treatment, sometimes the most important part.

How do we discover what is wanted? Observation is the key and sometimes the most difficult. This means using your five

88 Talking with Patients

senses, and the sixth sense called intuition without which the other five may mislead you. Look the patient in the eyes, because the eyes give away much that may never be said. Listen to what the patient says, how he says it, and particularly listen for what is not said. Feel for the patient's rapid pulse and look for the tremor of the hands that indicate anxiety. You should be able to smell fear, especially the fear of death, in the same way that you can taste the success of a good conversation.

Predicting the prognosis can be extremely difficult. Hence it is inadvisable to be too definite, best always to look on the bright side, and never to convey the impression of hopelessness; for without hope we die mentally if not physically. Predicting the prognosis is difficult because we have to assess the effect of the general health and age of the patient, the stage of disease, our experience of patients who have had a similar condition and the known natural history of that disease, as well as the patient's response to treatment. In all of these, we can be wildly wrong for a particular individual. Hence guarded answers do not indicate a refusal to be frank, but genuine ignorance. The patient, however, will expect truthful answers to his questions.

What disability, deformity or disfigurement will I have?
When will I get better and when can I return to work?
If the disease is likely to be fatal, how long have I got? How will I die? Will there be pain?

Predicting the prognosis is an art. The unlikely succumb, the doomed recover. Prognosis is something we learn about throughout life: it is rarely obvious and never without hope. Before answering the patient's request about prognosis ask yourself these questions.

● What must I tell the patient?

● How much of what I have found out should be told?

● What words should I use to convey the information?

● How much of what I intend to say will he understand?

● But, how will he know if I don't tell?

● How will he react? What will he do if I don't tell him?

Talking about diagnosis and prognosis 89

● Will he take my advice?
● How much pressure am I entitled to apply?

The patient of course asks similar questions of himself about the doctor, beginning with 'How much notice will he take of what I say to him?' Just as the nurse and doctor define the significant points in the patient's story, ignoring the seemingly irrelevant, so too the patient is selective in what he says. Sit on a bus and listen. Someone will talk about what he said to the doctor and how he survived. Health is good conversational material. As Querido (1959) has written: 'Whatever doctors may say to the contrary, their attitudes to patients under their care in hospital are publicly proclaimed by the way they act towards those patients'. Patients do not volunteer essential information of their psycho-social background which may have an unfavourable effect on their recovery from an illness, yet Querido (1959) listed six such items which can be discovered only by talking with the patient.

1. Bereavement by death of a member of the family or a close friend, particularly during the past year.
2. Serious illness or disability in anyone being cared for by the patient or living with the patient.
3. Problems with their own children.
4. Problems at work, actual or threatened.
5. Problems at home or with neighbours.
6. Other personal problems which the patient may be reluctant to mention.

When these six factors are taken into account and discussed openly and frankly the accuracy of predicting the prognosis increases substantially.

HOW TO REASSURE THE PATIENT

Most patients want reassurance as well as information about their illness and the future. Some require what might be termed 'reassurance in general', which can be provided in seven ways.

● Unspoken reassurance is given by the clinician's air of

90   Talking with Patients

authority, efficiency, and the optimism of other doctors and nurses. Reassurance flows from just sitting by the patient and showing confidence.

● Spoken words: to say 'there is nothing wrong with you' is trite; better to say 'there is nothing seriously wrong' or even 'no demonstrable disease has been found'. In the same way 'feeling rotten, today?' shows more understanding and shows sympathy than the more commonplace question 'how are you, today?'.

● The value of a complete examination of the ill patient should never be underestimated as an act of reassurance. For some patients this will be a new experience and may alarm; a few words of explanation will suffice to dispel new fears. A good bedside manner and personal attention works wonders.

● Restrict reassurance to what you know of the present condition. Do not talk about suspicions as though they were facts, but if the situation warrants it the patient can be told that things do not look serious when such is probable. If the illness is likely to be serious it is better to delay such opinion until there is sufficient evidence. It is sometimes worth diverting the conversation to an enquiry about the patient's job and hobbies if he persists in asking more than you can answer. In any case it is reasonable to say that you don't know at this stage. Do not use spurious explanations such as bad circulation, dry skin, night starvation, thin blood: they are unworthy of you.

People who don't think about themselves, don't worry. If the patient thinks about his condition, as indicated by the questions he asks, then he has worries – so deal with them. How much you tell depends on judgement from previous experience, but you have to be perceptive of unasked questions.

● An explanation, as guidance, about the likely future management of the patient is always appreciated. Explain what investigations need to be done and that you will tell the patient the results of these and what they mean. Outline what is involved in an investigation.

● One has to balance the risks of saying too much against those of saying too little. On some occasions, important and unpleasant information must be imparted at the first consultation even though 'bad news piece-meal' would be kinder. I

Talking about diagnosis and prognosis 91

recently saw a patient with metastatic malignant melanoma who was about to complete the mortgage for a new house. To say nothing about his future would have left his wife in an impossible financial position. The patient had to be told why he should not proceed with his mortgage.

● Finally, allow the patient the opportunity to talk to you alone and in privacy if he asks for this. Only under these conditions may you ever learn of the real and imaginary fears your patient has been harbouring. Always enquire if the patient has any special worries, and specifically ask if there is anything else that the patient would like to talk about, because such questions are in themselves reassuring. The aim must always be to make the patient feel that the situation, though serious, is not hopeless. A serious situation does not demand a long face; some humour is in order.

EXPECTATION

One lesson that rarely features in the undergraduate curriculum is the incurability of many disorders. The impression gained by nurses in training and medical students is the illusion that there is almost 100% potential for cure in all diseases, when in practice we have no cures for most of those numerous patients who suffer from cancer, heart disease, stroke, premature ageing, and psychiatric illnesses. So patients have to be made to understand what we can do and that nothing is easy in medical care.

An affluent society is an unhappy society. People's expectations are too great. Those who have money to spend expect to get what they want because 'money buys everything'. When they cannot get what they want they become bitter, angry, disbelieving. Those without money suspect that if they did have money they would receive better treatment.

Patent medicines and magic cures for intractable conditions are discussed on the radio, newspapers and magazines. Often the phrase 'Doctors don't understand' is added to make the message credible. Worse still, the speaker or writer may be referred to as 'doctor' (when all he possesses is a PhD in an unrelated subject), to increase the deception.

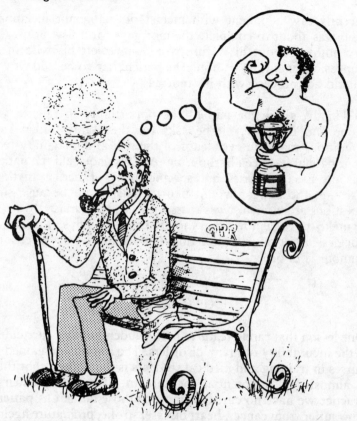

It is no wonder that patients believe that we don't know about 'breakthroughs' and 'advances' when we fail to take time to describe the factual state of our current knowledge. In talking with patients we have the chance to put things right. You will have to tell the patient how he will benefit. You have to 'sell' a line of treatment like a store salesman, but must not push the patient into blind acceptance; it should not be a 'hard sell' even if on some occasions that seems the only way to provide, apparently, a life-saving procedure. Convince the patient by explanation until he accepts readily and finds his decision emotionally satisfying. There is nothing wrong in saying 'You'll look better, feel better after treatment' by way of argument. Present the advantages, the good news, first before describing the disadvantages of therapy. And Hawkins (1967) wrote: 'Every doctor whatever his specialty, helps his patients simply

Talking about diagnosis and prognosis   93

by talking to them. Indeed, explanation and reassurance are essential for the care of every patient'.

The patient may already have firm convictions and expectations:

of what is 'normal',
of medical progress and miracles,
that money can buy health,
that everything has a physical basis,
that every illness is curable, and without risk,
that the unexpected rarely happens and will be unpleasant,
that the patient is not responsible for his illness and has no
   part to play in maintaining good health.

We have to understand how these have been arrived at and then correct any falsity.

THE TECHNIQUE OF EXPLANATION

We all know that diagnosis and prognosis have a bearing on treatment, but the two are so intimately related that certain points in the technique of explanation apply to both.

● Make it clear all the time what you are talking about (diagnosis, or investigations, or prognosis).

● Be sure to answer the basic questions that come into a patient's mind – the why, when, where?

● Be careful that the listener does not lose the thread in your longer sentences; if he does, start again, substituting shorter words and shorter sentences.

● Take care not to put unnecessary strains on your listener's memory. An important word, date, or dose should be written down.

● Follow a natural logical order in the conversation. Don't go

94 Talking with Patients

back and forth; you should sort out the sequences before talking and even when speaking should be thinking ahead.

● Avoid ambiguity at all costs unless this is deliberate and for good reason.

● Check that you have not missed something out; not just some vital detail such as the need for a blood transfusion or a general anaesthetic, but check on every expectation that your words raise. And what does it all amount to?

It pays to:

be concise,
make every word tell,
stay on firm ground,
avoid padding and irrelevancies,
watch the connotations of words and their pitfalls,
be careful with metaphors and figures of speech, if only to
    restrain the imagery from getting out of hand,
avoid repetition which has no special function,
use a summary at the end.

7

Talking about treatment

'Healing is a matter of time, but it is sometimes also a matter of opportunity.'

Hippocrates

Management of the patient's illness has often been described as 'getting things done', but it is only recently that the two-sided nature of the problem has been appreciated. The personal aspect of explaining treatment has now become the more important part instead of a mere incident to the technical process of getting things done.

Traditionally, the emphasis in medicine has always been placed on the technological aspect: the only problem with patients was to make them better. The art of persuading patients to help themselves actively is poorly done, yet the essence of therapy in hospital lies in the cooperation of three persons, the patient, the nurse and the doctor. This new thinking can only be effective if the patient agrees. Authority means more than just giving orders; it implies the acceptance of orders which determine what the patient is to do, or not to do, during treatment. A patient can only accept treatment if he understands it, and is able physically and mentally to comply. He will accept treatment if he believes that doing so is compatible with his interests and consistent with therapy for his illness. The key question for the patient submitting to treatment is 'Will it make me better?' (In social life we ask 'What's in it for me?'.)

Medicine has an authoritarian pattern of management. There is often no attempt to give the patient a feeling of security by informing him reliably of plans and prospects, and he is given no encouragement to participate in his treatment. He is at the mercy of 'decision-makers'. None of this need be so. Power with the patient is no more difficult than power over the patient; 'together we can get you better' is an easy approach, but you have to say so. As Hawkins (1967) has written 'What a doctor

96 Talking with Patients

says to his patients may be of far greater value than what he does for them'.

Many doctors and nurses challenge the idea that a patient wants any responsibility for his recovery. Some patients obviously do not, but a great many in my experience do and enjoy the sense of personal achievement in helping themselves; but all need guidance. The patient who accepts some responsibility will often want more. For instance, the value of early ambulation after operation is well recognised; not so much because it may prevent venous thrombosis in the legs or a little static mucus in the lungs, but because people get fit more quickly that way. The advice 'you can get out of bed when you like, you won't do any harm to your wound, and anyway you'll be happier going to the toilet rather than using a bedpan' can be coupled with the aside that 'Mr Smith was sitting out of bed four hours after his operation', as a spur to self-discipline and responsibility. The fact that Mr Smith is known to be over 70 years old will create the urge to do better. Children are different; give them the chance and they will be all over the place.

The encouragement to walk outside in the hospital grounds, to go to the hospital shop, and to give a hand with the distribution of food trays – not forgetting a pat on the back for a job well done – are important factors in allowing the patient responsibility for his immediate recovery. Patients who find that they can, after all, walk about quite well will inevitably wish to extend their activities. More than anything patients want the opportunity to appear cooperative and intelligent in the rather strange hospital environment. The patient has to know not only what is required of him, he needs to know why.

Maslow (1954) deplored the fact that whatever you do for people they are never satisfied, and put forward the concept of a hierarchy of needs at five different levels.

● Basically at the lowest level, physiological needs such as food, warmth and shelter.

● Safety needs, such as protection against threats and danger; the requirement is security, and familiarity with the known rather than the unknown.

● Social needs, such as affection and the feeling of belonging to a group.

Talking about treatment 97

● Esteem needs, the need for self-respect and the esteem of others, which implies recognition of status, personal attention, and the appreciation of one's abilities.

● The need for self-fulfilment, that is of self-creativeness.

It should be noted that everyone in hospital usually receives the first three on this list but not many patients can boast of the last two. Yet it is easy to fulfil all these needs by talking with patients.

MEDICAL TREATMENT

Medical treatment is largely about communication. You can write a prescription for a powerful drug and tell the patient to get it. But do you say when it should be taken? Three times a day. But before or after meals? What are the side-effects? Will it interfere with work, hobbies, pleasures, daily natural functions? Do we tell patients all this? Do we explain in simple terms? No, we don't. We presume they will read the label on the bottle. But the bottle containing tablets may provide little instruction and the name of the drug may be completely indecipherable. Little wonder that about half of all patients do not comply with their treatment and the annual 'spring clean' of the average domestic medicine cupboard reveals vast quantities of preparations, many expensive and some dangerous.

COMPLIANCE

What can we do to encourage patients to take the medicine we prescribe? First, to look at possible reasons for non-compliance; second, to consider the means by which patients can be helped to comply, that is by explanation and instruction.

There are many reasons for non-compliance but here is a list of the ten commonest.

● The medicine in itself may be unpleasant to take.

● It may produce nasty and unexpected side-effects.

98   *Talking with Patients*

● The medicine may have the wrong formulation: in Britain people expect tablets or a bottle of medicine (always for children), in France injections, in Italy suppositories, and so on. There are regional and national prejudices to be thought of and overcome.

● The patient may get better quickly, so does not bother, especially if he is adverse to taking drugs.

● Perhaps there is no immediate improvement in the illness and so faith is lost in that remedy.

● Neither the reasons for taking the medicine nor their importance may have been understood from the beginning.

● The patient may lack faith in the diagnosis and cannot believe that pills for a headache due to worry are likely to help.

● The patient may have too many tablets to take at different times each day, and so in confusion decides to abandon the lot.

● Warning advice from a 'friend'.

● No faith in the doctor.

In an attempt to increase the percentage of patients who will comply, three main methods have been tried with varying success.

Firstly, written instructions are given to each patient and it is ascertained that they are understood. A dietitian, for instance, does not try to inform patients by word of mouth alone, but provides a diet sheet and discusses this with the patient. As Fletcher (1980) has pointed out, people get clearer instruction when they buy a camera or transistor radio, than when they are given a life-saving antibiotic or cardiac drug. And that is not good enough. It must be acknowledged however that some associations (those for sufferers from diabetes, arthritis, and others) produce booklets that give sensible guidance to patients, as do many hospitals to those being admitted. But these provide general information and not the detailed knowledge required in specific therapy.

Secondly, the hospital pharmacy or the dispensing chemist provides a bag (for the medication) on which are printed

Talking about treatment 99

general instructions. At Hammersmith Hospital, the following are printed in red on the bag.

1. Read the directions carefully and give or take the exact recommended dose.
2. Complete the prescribed course – even if you do feel better.
3. Report any side effects you may have noticed.
4. Never share prescribed medicines with others.
5. If you are advised not to drink, drive or operate machinery while taking medicine – DON'T. It's dangerous.
6. If you're pregnant ask your doctor or pharmacist about any medicines you take.
7. Return unused prescribed or over-the-counter medicines to your pharmacist or throw them down the lavatory – not into a dustbin or on the fire.
8. Keep all medicines out of reach of children. Remember that to children brightly coloured tablets are just like sweets.
9. Never transfer medicines from the original container to another.
10. Never take medicines from unlabelled containers.
11. Treat all medicines with respect.

Regrettably, in an age of 'disposables', bags tend to get thrown away and not examined too closely – people think it is the contents that matter.

Thirdly, the doctor prescribing and the nurse at the clinic should take time to explain how, why and when medication should be taken. We now know that even in the best hands, with the simplest language and the most conscientious repetition, there is a 50% failure rate. Some doctors try to simplify the regime for taking tablets where many kinds are needed; others ask patients to bring the bottle with them at review to count the number of tablets remaining; others see their patients more often than necessary to try to check on compliance. But on the whole the results are disappointing. Perhaps the key is really that more time than most doctors can afford should be devoted to verbal explanation accompanied by precise written instructions. Certainly, too many people in talking with patients fail to introduce and discuss four important ideas: the concept of risk, that is to treat or not to treat; the real expectation of getting better naturally and without treatment or active medication; the

100 Talking with Patients

concept of cure or healing as a possibility or not; and finally the concept of amelioration or palliation.

Herxheimer (1977) has described a prompt sheet to be given to each individual patient. It consists of a list of questions which the patient may ask and for which answers should be provided. He argues that answers to questions which have been specifically asked are likely to be remembered and understood better than information delivered as a mini-lecture. The patient is encouraged to bring the sheet of questions to the follow-up clinic so that he may ask more questions which have been formulated between visits. The questions are grouped under five headings and reproduced here by permission.

1. *What is the name of the medicine?*
2. *What for and how?*
   > What kind of tablets are they and in what way will they help me?
   > Will I be able to tell if they are working?
   > How should I take them? Before or after meals, at night, with a lot of water?
3. *How important is the medicine?*
   > How important is it for me to take these tablets?
   > What is likely to happen if I do not take them?
   > What happens if I miss one dose? Should I take more the next time?
   > Are the tablets meant to treat the disease or relieve symptoms?
4. *Any side effects?*
   > Do the tablets cause any other effects that I should look out for? Do they ever cause any trouble? Should I let you know?
   > Is it all right to drive or climb heights while I am on the tablets? Are there any precautions to take?
   > Is it all right to take the tablets with other medicine I might need?
   > Will alcohol interfere with them?
   > Are there any foods I should avoid?
5. *How long for?*
   > How long will I need to continue with these tablets?
   > What should I do with any left over?
   > When will I see you again?

Talking about treatment 101

What will you want to know then?

Dunkelman (1979) has produced a check list for the simple procedures of investigation before an operation, of what is to be done and why. As a ward nurse she found that 50% of all patients were uninformed even though they had given consent to an operation. She, too, recommended verbal and written instructions, the latter to be presented first.

A record sheet given to the patient personally by the doctor or nurse will carry more weight than a 'patient package insert' already required by law in the USA when dispensing oral contraceptives, oestrogens and some other preparations. All printed material has one major defect: has the patient read and understood it? Patients need both written and verbal instructions, but above all a knowledge and understanding of disease, diagnosis and themselves which all takes time, but there are 10 points to remember.

● Stress the importance of the information.

● Use short words and short sentences. Choose words with care such that they mean the same to you as they do to the patient.

● Write down unfamiliar words such as medical terms, drugs and specific procedures.

● Categorise treatments where possible.

● Repeat words and sentences whenever you can.

● Give specific and detailed advice where necessary.

● Make concrete statements. Never be vague or abstract.

● Provide a calm and relaxed atmosphere for the occasion.

● Have a sympathetic, warm and responsive attitude when talking.

● Always encourage the patient to ask questions, and say that any not thought of at the time should be written down and brought to the next consultation. Promise to answer these questions frankly, however many there will be. If the explanation has been explicit and detailed, the patient is unlikely to ask

102   *Talking with Patients*

many questions. Often he will say 'You have covered all the questions I was going to ask', which is an important piece of information for you: the patient who prepares questions has thought about his disease and is more likely to comply in its management.

Moll and Wright (1978) believe that patients are good at remembering statements about diagnosis and that about 80% can recall explanation of symptoms. 'Less well remembered are statements to do with treatment and advice about what to do and when to do it. This may be because the doctor tends to become authoritarian; he decides what the treatment is to be, prescribes it, and gives instructions about how it must be carried out.' They note that the patient is rarely required to participate in treatment, may not listen to what is said, and may have difficulty in understanding and remembering unfamiliar language. For these reasons, Fletcher (1973) has advocated telling the patient about treatment before explaining the diagnosis. Both agree, however, that verbal and written instructions offer a better chance of the patient understanding what is required of him.

SURGICAL TREATMENT

Surgeons have a special relationship with their patients: they cut them. Although most of what has been written on medical treatment applies to patients who have a surgical operation, there are some added features to consider.

Under the heading of surgical treatment we can include those invasive investigative procedures that amount to a surgical operation anyway. Here, verbal explanations supplemented by written information will pay large dividends. The anaesthetist and the surgeon will see and talk with the patient beforehand and the patient will be required to sign consent. The patient will hear, see and do – the ideal requirements for remembering.

The doctor and nurse will need to explain several items.

● What will be done, who will do it, how will it be done, and when will it be done? Most patients are ignorant of the normal anatomy and physiology of their own bodies – not surprising

Talking about treatment 103

when you remember that a medical student spends two years on the subject and has to learn about 3000 new words. (This number could allow anyone to be reasonably fluent in a foreign language.) There is no need to use specific medical terms, but if you have to then write them down for the patient. A few minutes sketching the proposed operation is always appreciated. There is no need to go into detail but every reason to give a general outline. The first rule of every TV producer is this: don't say it, show it. It should be the same for us. The value of illustrations to demonstrate the diagnosis and operative treatment of his disease to a patient cannot be overstressed. The picture may tell the story more quickly and more effectively than words. The patient will obtain a visual impression to aid his understanding and this will reinforce what you tell him. There are three easy ways: simple diagrams, photographs, and pictures from books. The quickest by far is to draw something for the patient.

Diagrams have other advantages: they are easy to follow, they hold the attention, they can be built up by adding detail as you talk, they can be partly abstract to provide a concept which the patient can grasp quickly, and it is easier to locate the surgical condition on a body map. The patient can keep the drawing to study at leisure and to impress his relatives with. Yet you must be careful of the consequences. For instance, if a man has been advised to have his enlarged prostate removed, a simple diagram, showing obstruction to the bladder neck will explain the reason for the advice. But because the diagnosis was made by a finger in the rectum he may think that the operation will be done by the same route; he can hardly be blamed for thinking this. Hence a brief explanation of how the operation will be done is very necessary.

Pearson and Dudley (1982) asked 81 patients in a surgical ward about the function and location of parts of the gut, liver, gall bladder and pancreas: the majority did not know and some had quite erroneous ideas. These authors advised the routine use of duplicated simple line-diagrams to be handed to the patient during the explanation of the diagnosis and treatment. But a word of caution. Surgeons tend to describe diseases as though they were similar to everyday problems. Admittedly, some are mainly mechanical but comparison can give the wrong idea and make it all sound so easy when reality is otherwise.

104 Talking with Patients

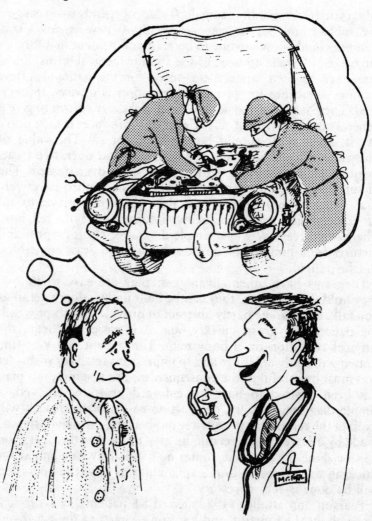

It is always advisable to discuss scars and the most likely complications (such as infection and bleeding), that is, to discuss the risks. Again no detail unless that is important for understanding or in helping the patient to come to a decision. In my experience, the commonest cause of acrimonious litigation is the failure to give the patient this elementary information. Even when information has been given verbally, a written note that the patient has been told should be recorded in the case

Talking about treatment 105

records. To keep out of the law courts, the surgeon must practise his art and the three C's: care, concentration and communication. If the consultant is to carry out the operation, this should be said; if not then the person who will should be introduced to the patient and his competence in the required procedure mentioned. This simple courtesy is frequently omitted in hospital so that afterwards patients do not know who did their operation, nor who to blame. Even if the operator is not in sole charge of the patient he should convey the feeling of authority and ability particularly during a ward round; by such means he can make the patient feel important and cement a personal relationship.

● What to expect afterwards. There are three versions which may differ markedly.

First, the surgeon's version, which must be a clear and precise description, based on his knowledge of the procedure and his experience of similar patients. Items that must be described to the patient and relatives are pain and its control, what an intravenous drip is, the need for antibiotics or other injections, whether the patient will return to the ward or stay in intensive care (some surgeons show their patients this area before operating), and whether the patient will receive supportive procedures such as tracheostomy and artificial ventilation. (The word drip means nothing to most patients; what about drain – pipes and guttering?) The surgeon will tell the patient that he will see him in the anaesthetic room immediately before operation and afterwards in the ward when he regains consciousness. He will also spend some time telling the patient the result of the operation and be willing to talk with relatives if the patient wishes.

Second, the nurse's account, which may dwell more on bedpans and bed baths and the fact that she will be there to care for the patient afterwards. In my view a nurse is entitled to answer questions put to her by the patient about his operation, to the best of her ability, but should not volunteer information; that is the surgeon's job and a second opinion is likely to confuse and alarm a patient rather than reassure. The nurse should not make too light of even a minor procedure; the majority of operations are minor for an experienced surgeon, but all are major for the patient.

106 *Talking with Patients*

Third, the account given by the patient in the next bed, which may be frightening or comforting. To a large extent the general morale in a ward plays a large part in allaying anxiety; the higher the morale the more comforting the unsolicited information.

● The anaesthetist will visit the patient in the ward, not just to make a physical examination and prescribe premedication, but to tell the patient his name, who he is, who will be giving the anaesthetic and how it will be given, and to repeat some of the information already provided by the surgeon. A few minutes of general chat is useful because the patient will recognise the anaesthetist's face and voice again in the anaesthetic room just before the operation, will readily obey instructions during the wake-up period ('open your mouth, take a big breath', are common instructions as well as 'Your operation is over, everything will be fine'), and will be comforted by a familiar voice in the recovery room.

There is now good evidence (Egbert, Battit, Welch, and Bartlett, 1964) that simply by talking with the patient beforehand, the anaesthetist plays an important part in the patient's recovery: there is less pain and fewer 'pain-killers' are required, the patient is out of bed sooner, and discharged from hospital earlier. To call this a placebo effect is wrong: it is simply common courtesy. If a patient knows what to expect he will understand what is required of him and cooperate. There is also good evidence that patients who are advised to stop smoking at this time will do so. The coincidence of a suitable opportunity and personal advice is far more effective than all the public advertising that smoking is bad for your health.

● Two questions should always be asked before operation and asked separately: Have you any questions you wish to ask about the operation or the anaesthetic? Is there anything else worrying you? The answers to these often reveal hidden fears which can so easily be put right. Fears grow when left unattended; the best way to deal with fear is to put the record straight early on.

Patients with fear fall into roughly three groups. There are the terrified, who are restless, sleepless and tearful. They worry about minor details of the operation, require repeated assurance,

Talking about treatment 107

and benefit from tranquillisers before and after operation. They may still be anxious after a successful procedure even though they express gratitude and admiration for all the attention received. Then there are the moderately afraid, who have realistic fears but will adapt to the prospect of some pain. The third group is those with minor fears, who appear relaxed and uncomplaining and are often known as good patients. Some, however, have never faced up to the prospect of an operation or have refused to do so. These patients may later become moody, uncooperative and even belligerent. Nothing seems to go right for them.

To add to all these there is a procedure which Bennett (1979) calls 'stripping': the process whereby 'a new patient is stripped of the outward signs of individuality by the removal of clothes and personal possessions including the various bits and pieces most people need if they are to look their best when facing the world. The new patient is assigned to a hard and unusually high bed, possibly one amongst 20 or 30 others'. He becomes an anonymous patient in an anonymous ward. Worse will follow. A young nurse comes and asks questions, so that patients in adjacent beds may gather more details than his neighbours ever did. A young doctor follows to ask about personal habits and family relationships in addition to purely medical questions – more a public hearing than a private conversation. Little wonder the patient has become conditioned to anxiety about his operation, which he fears may be just as public, and suffers loss of sleep in consequence (Murphy, Bentley, Ellis and Dudley 1977).

In return, the hospital provides the security of regular food and water, protection from the elements, freedom from work, care for hygiene and health. Under such unnatural conditions the patient may suffer severe strain which goes unrecognised by all about him. One patient will read, listen to the radio and withdraw into himself; another will make the most of the opportunity to explore new surroundings. Both, however, will suffer from what Desmond Morris (1977) calls the 'stimulus struggle' for survival. The patient who has been used to the give-and-take of conversation with his mates at work, the pressure of his job, and the influence of friends will miss such intellectual and physical stimulation.

If the stimulus of being in hospital is too weak, the patient will overcome this by creating unnecessary problems for

108 Talking with Patients

himself, which he can solve, or over-reacting to a normal stimulus, such as pain or discomfort, or inventing novel activities, or magnifying ordinary events; sometimes he will do all these. If the stimulus in hospital is too strong, then the patient's normal response will be dampened down. The patient also has an illness, with plenty of time to think about it, so quite naturally very simple worries are magnified.

It is in this environment that communication with the patient has to operate. No wonder the patient is unable to concentrate and will understand only about half of what is said, let alone ask the right questions or grasp the answers. It takes a little time for the new patient to settle down in a ward of 30 and to become one of the community; denial of this need to belong to a group is an important seed of discontent. Yet the patient wants companionship which he can and will obtain readily from other patients, if not from staff, but it takes time.

● In an emergency it may be possible to talk to a patient only briefly. The patient must take your word on trust, but soon afterwards he will expect answers to four questions.

What did you do?
Why did you do it?
What did you find?
What does it mean?

They are simple, direct and clear questions. The answers, in the same terms, will satisfy most patients. Even so, it is worthwhile to talk with the patient again at a later date in case he is not clear in his own mind about the why and what of his treatment. Few patients wish to know how the operation was done, and rarely is it asked as a serious question; a fairly light-hearted reply will suffice.

After operation the patient will expect to be told when he may get out of bed, when he can go home, when he can return to normal activities, when he will be seen again, and how his own general practitioner fits into the scheme of things. Simple explanations are important and they should not be left so the patient has to ask. For instance, if the patient has been provided with a sling after an operation on his hand, explain why. 'The sling is to hold your hand up without effort. It will help you to

Talking about treatment 109

have less pain and less swelling than if your hand is below the level of your elbow, but do keep moving your fingers. Better still, you will get sympathy from your friends and are likely to get a seat on a crowded bus. Wear it for the next three days, but take it off at night when you're in bed. Please bring it back again when we meet.' Explain everything you can; patients expect it, welcome it, and are grateful. If an instruction sheet is available, make sure the patient has a copy and that he reads it. Encourage him to ask questions for clarification, by saying 'It's your hand so look after it, and if you have any queries just ask'.

● If the operation is to be done under local anaesthesia special care is needed in what is said and what is done, irrespective of whether the patient is sedated. Operating theatres can be noisy places, so the first thing is to limit the unnecessary noise of moving instruments about, people coming and going, loud voices. This requires training and a constant awareness that the patient is not deaf.

In talking, choose your words with care: do not use words which have unpleasant connotations such as blood, needle, syringe, scissors, knife, and many others. If the surgeon requires a particular suture it is just as easy and kinder to say 'May I have a five-o-silk with a twenty millimetre end, and it should be triangular' as 'I'll sew up with a five-o-silk suture on a twenty millimetre cutting needle'. The difference for the patient over-hearing what is said, as indeed he must, is enormous. If the patient is talking with the nurse sitting beside him, he will ignore the first statement, but will invariably halt his conversation for the second. Of course, everyone in the theatre team must be in the know. It is a minor disaster when a newcomer translates the surgeon's carefully worded request into blunt language, starting with 'Do you mean ...'. To anyone who operates on children under local anaesthesia, the therapeutic effect of talking is a continual wonder. Once the local anaesthetic has taken effect, a skillful nurse can divert the child's atttention completely in a few minutes. There is so much to talk about – school, teachers, holidays, hobbies, family and home life – the list is endless. Much the same applies to adults who often are very nervous and do not have that simple trust displayed by children.

110   *Talking with Patients*

● When an invasive type of investigation is being done under a local anaesthetic, such as an arteriogram, it is important that the patient is kept well informed during the procedure. He will have been told, perhaps formally, what will be done, how and why but now he should be told conversationally what is going on. The conversation will switch from observed facts to generalities and back again. The patient will expect to be told the result of the special investigation; it is a good idea to say at the time what has been found and to repeat the same information later when the procedure is finished and everyone has relaxed. If you find nothing abnormal, say so. Do not say 'there's nothing to worry about'. There is a virture in showing the relevant x-rays, for instance, and pointing out the important features. It is not necessary to give a lecture, but rather to treat the patient as your equal, to show kindness and respect for his intelligence. Some patients will make apt remarks and put your information in more pithy and everyday language than you do; try to remember their words and use them on a future occasion. Patients do have faith in doctors and nurses, they do have a sense of purpose; they want both of these to be recognised by their medical attendants, but will not tolerate deception. 'Oh what a tangled web we weave when first we practise to deceive', and the first result of this web is the patient's loss of confidence in us.

When you realise that 50% of all patients, medical and surgical, are in hospital for five days or less and so do not have time enough to get to know the many nurses and doctors they meet, it should become clear that important information must be given to the patient as soon as it is known. Time is on no-one's side. So talk now.

8

The fatal illness

'You cannot demonstrate an emotion or prove an aspiration.'
Morley

Cancer, dying, bereavement are often the ingredients of the last illness, the fatal illness. The three subjects are considered together because they have one important aspect in common; they are all highly emotive. Talking about them is rarely easy. We are all in three parts: the body, the mind, and the spirit; of this trinity any one part may degenerate or die first. Dying is not always an instantaneous affair as many patients seem to think. Yet, doctors and nurses tend to be off-hand when the subject is raised by the patient. Staff are embarrassed, understandably so, by the questions the patient may ask, and by their personal failure to cure.

Some people fail to recognise that death is inevitable sooner or later, because no-one is immortal, and that the time spent talking to dying patients may be longer than expected but it is time well spent. The essence of the relationship between doctor and patient should be of trust and privacy. On both sides. The patient trusts the doctor and the doctor trusts the patient. 'I won't let you down' can be spoken by both. Medicine aims to improve the quality of life, not prolong it. This simple concept has led to confusion because when treatment has failed to cure disease and the patient is going to die, the doctor and nurse feel they too have failed. They do not recognise that the patient requires another form of treatment which is time-consuming and that they should, through training and ability, be in a position of power to give this service. When all medication has failed and there is only good nursing and loving care left, talking assumes a new importance: it becomes therapy and the good talker takes over. And the best of these will be the one who can use his imagination and ingenuity while being exquisitely sensitive to the need of the moment.

112 *Talking with Patients*

8.1 The attractive speaker

1. Has a pleasant voice that can be heard easily.
2. Uses memorable and colourful phrases.
3. Has clear diction.
4. Looks alive and interested.
5. Uses appropriate gestures, quite naturally.
6. Varies his rate and rhythm of speaking.
7. Has a good command of English but uses words appropriate to his audience.
8. Uses pauses to good effect.
9. Has a sense of timing, an individual style.
10. Has an ease of manner, a sense of humour, patience and understanding in the way he converses.

TALKING ABOUT DYING

It is a continual matter of amazement to me that patients with serious and prolonged illness are not only unprepared for death, they do not believe it will occur. They expect doctors to work miracles and never seem to realise the living miracle that they have been for the past few years when death has seemed inevitable. Because of medical treatment? Perhaps. Despite medical treatment is often the true answer.

So, the problem of how to prepare the patient for death is a real one. An unpleasant duty which should not be dodged. When death seems inevitable, the doctor and nurse have great moral and social responsibilities. As Bennett (1979) has written 'Looking after a dying person involves caring; and often more than if he is going to live.'

Fletcher (1973) asked 'Why don't we talk about dying?' and listed six reasons why we do not.

● Dying represents failure for both doctors and nurses and so both feel embarrassed, guilty, and not keen to talk. We would much rather talk of our succcesses; even though an outsider might consider the achievement of a painless and peaceful death

The fatal illness 113

a considerable success when this seemed unlikely, we still recognise it as failure to survive. The cost of a short-lived and miserable survival is seldom compared by doctors and nurses with a quick painless death, even though this comfort is frequently offered to the patient's relatives.

● Explaining death to the patient is costly in time and emotionally demanding. The patient's family become involved and want to talk, so even more interview time is required.

● There is poor training in medicine for the job of talking about dying, yet the obvious answer – to enlist the help of the clergy, social worker, hospice nurse or even the relatives – is seldom considered until late.

● It is difficult to know how much to tell.

● It is easy to leave the task to someone else.

● The patient is often depressed, resentful and angry, so that the task is made even more demanding emotionally than it might have been. To be blamed by the patient for his probable demise, when you have expended time and energy to hold back the inevitable, is a bitter pill to have to swallow before getting on with the job of supplying physical and moral comfort.

In addition, many people forget that dying is in two parts: the moment of death and the run-up to it. At the moment of death we all will want privacy, quiet, familiar surroundings, the love of relatives and some spiritual warmth: all of these are best at home especially if death is peaceful as it generally is. In the run-up to death, which may be weeks or months away, the patient's disease may no longer be treated actively because it is beyond that, but he may have pain. There are three kinds of pain: physical, social and spiritual. The physical pain can be relieved by drugs, but the feeling of being an outcast, lonely, frightened and depressed demands good, frequent and effective talking. Mother Theresa in the slums of Calcutta, surrounded by the poor, diseased, hungry and overcrowded was asked, 'What is the greatest misfortune in this life?'. Her reply: 'loneliness'. We forget that the seriously ill and the dying can be lonely in a crowded ward. They need more talk and attention, not less, than others.

114 *Talking with Patients*

8.2 We talk to

1. Identify ourselves to others.
2. Create images: we think in language.
3. Transfer our thoughts.
4. Establish a relationship.
5. Banish loneliness and fear.
6. Reassure ourselves.

Knowledge, skill and experience may not help much, but some planning will. Moreover, the 'inverse-care law' states that those most in need of care, such as the chronic sick and the dying, often do not get it; modern medicine is geared to cure.

PLANNING YOUR TALK

Although planning has been discussed earlier in a different context, here we have to consider 12 aspects which concern the seriously ill. The speaker will be acting as an informant and confidant. The 12 questions to ask yourself are given below.

● What to say? To some extent this depends on how much the patient already knows. If you have talked with him before, you will have a good general idea; if you have not then you may have to probe with some questions first. Questions should be put with understanding, compassion, and a great deal of tact, but they must be asked.

Where does the patient get his medical knowledge from? From medical textbooks and journals? Most unlikely. Admittedly, most public libraries carry books on health, disease, doctoring and nursing for anyone to borrow and read. The output of popular medicine for the public by other means is continuous and vast: the *Readers Digest*, daily newspapers, women's magazines, a weekly series on television and radio; and a great deal emanates from relatives and fellow patients, which may be wildly inaccurate and sometimes alarming.

So there are many sources of information; some accurate,

The fatal illness 115

others grossly inaccurate in the quality of information supplied. Many feature articles are written by non-medical people whose research of a new subject, new angle, new treatment is superficial and lacking in understanding. Few articles present the advantages and disadvantages of a new drug or new operation, believing the general public not to be interested in such details. An ill patient, however, is in quite a different category. Like a drowning man he clutches at straws and hopes for speedy cure. In addition to a limited knowledge of disease, the patient may have unduly high expectations from therapy and a lack of understanding of his own anatomy and bodily functions. All three factors largely determine the patient's attitude to his illness and to those who attend him, including his relatives.

However, if you listen the patient will often indicate what he wants to know. He may well tell you the diagnosis.

There are two conflicting views often put forward by the healthy, who are really in no position to be dogmatic; the belief that everything in medicine is black or white with no grey area between is naive and widespread. The first view is that a doctor has no right to withhold knowledge of a fatal disease, and so the patient must be told. The second is that a doctor has no right to tell the patient everything about his illness, especially if he does not want to know. It may well be that the majority of patients want to be told the truth about themselves and for various reasons: for peace of mind, to help in understanding illness, to help in planning follow-up appointments, for planning their own future, family finance and religious matters. But it is arrogant nonsense to insist that every patient is told. Many patients do not want confirmation of doubts. If they have a fatal cancer yet continue to remain in good health, then as time passes it is easier to believe that things will be alright. These patients are happy with their ignorance. To confirm fatal cancer in a patient who does not want to know will kill his spirit, and he will probably die sooner; his will to live has been defeated. We presume that knowing the truth, the full facts, always brings out the best in people. In practice it often has the opposite effect.

● How to say it? Introduce the subject gradually but do not be woolly in what you say. There is no need to be blunt, indeed

116 Talking with Patients

you should rarely be blunt, but the patient must be clear about what you say and the words you use. If you have established a good relationship with the patient, a normal conversational-type of informality will do well.

● When to say it? The patient often provides the lead. Sometimes the subject will be mentioned to a nurse first who may discover quite fortuitously that a patient has no idea of the seriousness of his condition. The good nurse will pass that information to the doctor-in-charge so that this ignorance can be corrected. At other times it will be raised during conversation. For instance, I had one patient who, after the usual chatty pleasantries, suddenly said, 'I suppose I will die of my cancer'. My reply was 'Yes, you will ... You're lucky in a way. I don't know how I will die. It may be violent. Yours won't be, and it will be painless'. We then went on to discuss the family and how they would manage after the patient's death. There was no embarrassment. A little weeping, yes, but a good cry is no bad thing. The patient wanted to talk and felt better for it. Talking always makes bad news better.

Never delegate to a junior what is your duty to do. Never, that is, unless you are confident that the other will do as well if not better than you. If you are not competent to deal with a situation find someone who is and introduce him to the patient. Say why you are doing this, for example because he is the expert in the field.

It takes courage to sit down and talk bad news, courage on both sides, but courage and bravery never go out of fashion. You may have to ask yourself: What can I say now? What can be left to the future? The patient has a right to talk about death; the doctor and nurse must listen and give the patient the opportunity to talk.

● Where to say it? An open ward is hardly a good place in which to discuss details. If the patient can be moved to a quiet room, talking in privacy especially if relatives will be interviewed at the same time will be appreciated. In spite of modern curative medicine and computers, communication with patients is a frail and difficult business. The least you can do is to provide the best possible conditions for face-to-face talking.

● Who to tell? In my view, if the patient wishes to know details

The fatal illness 117

of his fatal condition he should be told first. He can be asked if he would like you to tell his spouse or relatives. If he does not want others to know, this request should be honoured. It may be worth discussing the value of others knowing, and pointing out that they probably do know or at least suspect already. It is usually helpful that husband and wife should know the bad news so that they can discuss it openly, frankly, and plan accordingly. Certainly this makes things easier for the medical attendants.

When relatives are interviewed it is only courteous to provide a cup of tea, to enquire about transport home, to allow them to talk privately to those nursing the patient, to explain what is likely to happen and that you are available for further talks if required. This interview, like all others, should be a dialogue, and time must be allowed for that. It is the main chance to anticipate grief and to point out that death is not a medical rarity.

● How much detail to disclose? Honesty and tact are not mutually exclusive. The direct question 'Have I got a fatal cancer?' does not demand a direct answer. You have to use your imagination and be realistic. The immediate answer must depend on the patient's own prior knowledge and the degree of urgency. Do not take your talking out of context: the very ill patient and the very well patient should receive different replies. You have to weigh up the question and reply appropriately.

It will be necessary to discuss the four D's: disability, deformity, disfigurement and death. But not all at once. It will also be necessary to discuss the fear of pain, loneliness, depression and sleeplessness.

● How many visits will be required to get the whole message across? Usually more than one.

● What is the order of priorities? What should be discussed first? The good news first, always. The patient's fear of disablement may be greater than his fear of dying.

● What are the features to concentrate on? Prognosis or diagnosis? Which will help this patient to understand his condition and his future?

● What should be written down for the patient?

118   *Talking with Patients*

● Will illustrations help understanding? Will anecdotes of other patients help?

● What help does the patient require from a clergyman, social worker, visitors, family? If I were the patient, what would I like now? The first principle of an information system is to communicate salient facts to the people who are in a position to act on them. If you agree, you have to tell others what help you want. You have to learn to recognise a problem and then deal with it as soon as you can; there is no advantage in waiting.

You have to develop a certain confidence in talking about death and dying – the two are not the same and the distinction should be made: more people by far are afraid of the process of dying rather than the state of death itself.

Enlist the trust and support of the priest, social worker, psychologist, hospice nurse, visitors and anyone else who may be helpful in management, but one person must be in charge to control and coordinate the team effort. In industrial practice it has been found that the maximum 'span of control' is about six: beyond that number there are difficulties of communication and contact. The same is probably true in medicine although it is quite common to have more than six people concerned with the welfare of one patient. On the whole, the fewer the better.

There are also self-help groups, usually lay-people who can provide important instructions for the patient and speed his return to normal living: the local stoma care, mastectomy, stroke and other asssociations are usually known to the social worker but you must ask the patient's permission before seeking help. Some patients definitely do not want others to know of their condition.

We can create mutual understanding and confidence only by talking and doing. In most enterprises there has to be something tangible, something to show to others, by which to gauge success. But in talking with the dying there seems to be no easy method of assessment. So how can one tell if one has done a good job? In two ways: by measuring performance against an assumed professional standard, and by the quality and quantity of letters of appreciation from relatives and friends of the deceased.

The fatal illness 119

THE PATIENT'S ATTITUDE TO HIS DIAGNOSIS

Brewin (1977) has written about the way in which patients react to the news that they have cancer. His classification of attitudes applies just as pointedly to all patients on first hearing the diagnosis of their illness, whether this be of serious import or of little consequence.

There are at least ten different responses to be recognised. The patient who learns that he has a fatal illness reacts in a recognisable way. Kubler-Ross (1969) has pointed out that patients pass through five stages of emotion when they hear the bad news: shock and denial of the diagnosis is followed by anger which may be vented on the doctor, nurse, relative or other patients. This may be followed by a period of bargaining to buy time which leads to the depression of knowing that such cannot be. Finally there is acceptance of the likely outcome: previous experience of a death in the family may help to mould and direct the patient's attitude. Some patients may skip a stage, some never come to accept the inevitable.

Patients clearly do have fears when they hear the diagnosis. People are frightened of death, are frightened of doctors and nurses at times, certainly are frightened by monitoring gadgetry, but mainly frightened of the future.

● *The needy.* Assurance that the condition is not serious and the outlook not hopeless is the desperate desire of this patient. Once the doctor or nurse, with authority and complete confidence, has given this assurance the patient may not wish or even be able to listen to any further information. Further talks, when the patient is in a more receptive frame of mind and calmer, are always necessary; not just to reinforce the original reassurance but to get across to him what the diagnosis really means and what his treatment entails.

The patient may accept the diagnosis in silence. On such occasions it is necessary to ask him questions so that the clinician can discover if the patient really understands. The phlegmatic acceptance may be because the patient is naturally taciturn or a slow-thinker, and so his interest must be aroused before he will listen to advice. Some, of course, are excessively nervous, even terrified and unable to speak, but will behave differently at a second consultation. Beware of the patient who

120   Talking with Patients

is as cool as new sheets; he sometimes needs reassurance, explanation and instruction more than anyone.

● *The optimist*: Often the aggressively cheerful optimist makes a great effort to reject mentally any bad news. This patient will be angry, upset, and even abusive if he is forced to listen to a blunt statement that he is seriously ill. A tactful approach always pays off, perhaps spread over many visits. But the real question is: should the patient's optimism be destroyed, and to what extent? Clearly the patient with a fatal illness and a young family who is about to apply for a house mortgage has to be dissuaded from leaving behind impossible debts for his wife. Straight talking is only fair, and is imperative. What about the older person who has made his will, whose dependents have been catered for? Well why bother? Some doctors and nurses insist that patients must be told everything, a form of ideology. But on the whole ideologies are disappointing substitutes for common sense.

Some patients become so talkative that they will not allow the doctor or nurse to proceed. Others will become argumentative, disputing every statement, questioning every opinion. It is sometimes difficult for the medical attendant not to get rattled and heated in return, but it is a grave error. Do not argue, but wait for an opportunity to explain. Some patients are pompous, filled by their own importance and a little knowledge, so that they show their lack of real understanding; but they are susceptible to flattery.

● *The 'Give me the full facts', patient* often does not mean what he says. The demand represents an attempt to appear adult in a complex and difficult personal situation. So speak with care. A series of questions, to try to find out why he wants 'the full facts' is in order and advisable (the answers may reveal that the full facts would destroy his spirit, utterly) before attempting to explain a single detail. However, where the diagnosis is clear, unequivocal, and not serious the patient should always be told at the first opportunity. The patient's reaction is frequently one of relief. Where the disease is serious it is kinder to provide information piece-meal.

● *The relaxed and philosophical patient* is confident that he is in the best hands, that everything possible is being done for his

The fatal illness 121

benefit. He is not keen to discuss diagnosis nor prognosis. 'I leave it all to you doctor' is the attitude, but somehow we have to impart a little information which he will note and use. The patient may live from day-to-day but we have a duty to point to tomorrow. Brewin recorded that in his experience these patients form by far the largest group in the UK, particularly when dealing with cancer. They are the most satisfying people to deal with, but that is no reason to neglect communication of facts which may be important to the patient and his family. The patient may have undisclosed fears which only surface after gentle probing. Good timing and irrelevant small talk about nothing in particular may open the flood gates to a very different situation. Remarkably often the patient's fears are groundless, his worries highly soluble, and covert misery can be turned to overt happiness at a stroke. To do this you have to probe, gently, repeatedly.

● *The tense and suspicious patient* is more of a problem. He badly needs information. Set time aside, sit down and chat. Start off with generalisations, about disease, medicine, your own circumstances or specialty, then get down to the details of his diagnosis, his treatment, his prognosis, without giving a black picture. Discuss the side effects of treatment as well as visiting hours. It is rarely necessary to tell the patient everything, rather to give him something to think about and to prompt questions which he can mull over and ask when you see him again. Such patients are often considered morose and difficult in a ward; they can be won over, and changed out of all recognition in fifteen minutes of listening and talking. Sometimes listening is the more important, and that's where judgement and experience really count.

● *The disbeliever* is the patient who cannot or will not accept that illness has come to him. Even when the evidence is laid before him, he is unable to believe it. 'There must be some mistake' is his reply.

The attitude of this patient may become ill-mannered, even abusive, to the doctors and nurses attending him. He will blame others for his condition. Or he may produce a negative response, listening to all that you tell him, and then declaring that he will not accept the diagnosis and will seek advice elsewhere (in my experience few do). Such patients require

122 *Talking with Patients*

understanding rather than sympathy, and for them a talk with their relatives is always worthwhile, if only to insure that he cannot state truthfully that he was not told the diagnosis.

● *The 'favoured-treatment' patient* accepts the diagnosis without understanding and expects to receive preferential treatment immediately. The patient may be angry when not given a private room if admitted to hospital, or kept waiting at a follow-up appointment. In some, this is a form of escapism from the reality of disease, but in many it is a form of selfishness born of fear. Such patients require a disproportionate amount of one's time if a serious attempt is to be made to comprehend the reasons for their behaviour.

● *The harassed patient* may be unable to make up his mind to accept the diagnosis and will return asking for further confirmatory tests. It is easy to accede to such requests, but dangerous. The clinician may end up with too much information! There is solace and security in multiple investigations, but regrettably deception for self and patient too.

● *The passive patient* accepts the diagnosis, becomes dependent on others, enjoys the role of an invalid often for secondary gain, and accepts illness as a habit. This patient may complain to hospital authorities, the Department of Health, the local Member of Parliament, the Head of State, that his new symptoms have not been attended to or that he is receiving inadequate treatment. The amount of extra work such a patient can cause is unbelievable until you experience it.

● *The hopeless and helpless patient* is different. He will often be depressed, rarely feel well, never appear cheerful or grateful, and continually mourns his bad fortune. He is a 'pain in the neck' to everyone with whom he comes in contact.

COMFORT

'To cure sometimes, to relieve often, to comfort always' is the traditional concept of the doctor's role in society. But how to do so, that's the nub. Advances in therapy allow more cures and more relief of suffering, but the comfort? It was never taught formally at nursing or medical school, because traditionally

The fatal illness 123

students have been left to develop skill through the untutored observation of senior staff at ward rounds and out-patient clinics, and left to practise on their own with neither surveillance nor constructive criticism. Failure to teach explicitly the sort of thing to say, when and how, no longer meets the obligation of doctors and nurses to their patients. It is not so much that patients are now more demanding, but that social, family and environmental factors, and problems at work, play a larger part in the cause of ill-health than formerly (or, at least, are now more generally recognised). No longer is grandma or the priest available to confide in. So how can we provide the comfort?

First, the patient will want to know about diet, work, smoking, alcohol, exercise and hobbies (especially in the case of judo or even yoga) so why not anticipate these unasked questions? The answers do not have to be written down because they are usually remembered. The answers can be slipped in, without embarrassment, in describing the medical management of the patient's condition. All this adds to the patient's confidence that his doctor understands, is sympathetic, interested and has a wide and knowledgeable experience of the patient's disease. It requires, from the doctor, little effort but much thought, some knowledge of human nature, and the ability to talk freely with his patient.

Second, he will expect complete confidentiality and be comforted by that knowledge, which may well have to be stated openly. Patients are immensely discomfited by the hearing of their own troubles from a third party. So never gossip about patients however astonishing their news.

Third, patients need someone to talk with, to confide in, to go into intimate details with, someone whom they can trust. As Corneille wrote, 'By speaking of our misfortunes we often relieve them'. Even in a 30-bedded ward it is easy to be lonely and worried. There is no such thing as equality; some patients need more comfort than others. The lonely, the frightened, and children must have frequent assurance and explanations. They may not completely understand all that is said, but the mere presence of a doctor or nurse is in itself reassuring; this 'coded' message of reassurance is passed to parents and visitors, a kind of domino effect. In this manner, fears and doubts are dispelled as soon as they form.

124 *Talking with Patients*

Fourth, friendship provides comfort. Most would agree that a deep and lasting friendship is a precious and enriching experience, but the number of true friends we make in a lifetime is very small. Friendship emerges in a gradual way, as a relationship of sharing something and a commitment to the same goal. It is a form of companionship which patients value but do not often receive. It does not, and perhaps should not, require the doctor or nurse to be involved emotionally in the patient's illness, but there is nothing wrong in showing your feelings.

Fifth, an infusion of what Cousins (1976) called the positive emotions of 'love, hope, faith, laughter, and the will to live' helps.

Sixth, the personality of the doctor is a powerful form of treatment, but few can change their personality. What doctors and nurses can do is to develop an ease of manner, a sense of humour, patience, understanding, and above all confidence in talking with patients. The other qualities, of authority and expertise, come a long way down the list of the patient's needs. Those with real ability to converse will be guided by the four C's: consideration for others, confidence in the diagnosis and the therapeutic management, courage to do the right thing, and ability to obtain the cooperation of the patient.

Seventh, the preservation of high morale in the individual patient, the staff, and in the ward generally. With high morale almost anything can be achieved; without it, very little. When morale goes, people cannot think, never mind clearly or imaginatively; life itself is threatened and self-preservation comes first.

Lastly, a progress report is always appreciated. Progress may be good or slow, but never bad. There is great comfort in knowing, and being told, that you are doing well. The progress report should be reinforced by gestures that convey affection (a smile will do) and by physical contact (a touch on the arm or shoulder).

TALKING WITH THE BEREAVED

If you can not come to terms with the idea of your own death then probably you will not be able to satisfy the psychological needs of your dying patient or the bereaved relatives. This does

The fatal illness 125

not mean that you should be afraid to show your own feelings. It is not only babies who cry. We all get depressed and discouraged by terminal illness and our failure to serve and save those entrusted to our care.

If relatives take part in the care of the patient they tend to grieve less. Shared care is satisfying and relieves anxieties as well; in films the expectant father is always put to work to provide plenty of hot water although we never learn what it will be used for. No two bereavements are the same and so regaling the bereaved with details of your own experience is usually unhelpful; your own experience of death will have sharpened your perception so that you see things not otherwise seen and will help you to appreciate the other person's feelings, but don't ever say 'I know how you feel', because you may not. One of the saddest phrases to hear is 'If only I had ...'. You may have to provide comfort and an instant opinion, supported by sound arguments, why action by the relative could not have changed the outcome. Not an easy task.

Don't be afraid of talking to the bereaved about the dead; it is the body that will be buried, not the memories. A good conversational opening about your own (deceased) patient is 'I wish I had know him better. Tell me about him'. The bereaved relative wants to talk, so let him. Sometimes the dam breaks and there are floods of tears: don't be too embarrassed to put an arm round the patient or to offer a tissue. Crying is therapeutic and oddly satisfying. Oh, that people would cry more.

Grief can lower the threshold of tolerance in any household; what would be a small upset in a happy family can become a major disaster in a broken one. A loving wife or husband can be turned into a miserable and embittered widow or widower by the tragedy. Those closest to the bereaved have to bear the brunt of their pain which may be expressed in a hurtful manner. Moreover, the faith of even the most committed Christian may be shattered by grief and so offer no comfort.

Many towns now have bereavement counselling run as a voluntary service. Councillors can help the bereaved relatives of your patient in many ways. They offer practical help (particularly for the first few days) such as answering the door or telephone, doing the shopping, being a companion when the relative goes for the death certificate, arranging the funeral, and will fend off well-wishers who do not realise that bereavement

126   Talking with Patients

is exhausting and that the bereaved must be allowed to spend some time alone. The councillor and the hospice nurse will often go to the funeral or at least babysit if there are young children in the family.

Finally, there is the problem of the bereaved who will have to cope single-handed with job, home and family. He needs a plan and help. He needs to talk about both to someone who will listen.

TALKING WITH STAFF

The question of how doctors and nurses cope with their own feelings while looking after the dying is seldom raised. A survey among nurses in the USA (Cheyney, 1980) disclosed personal emotional difficulties in caring for the following, in increasing order of acceptance: a young child, an adolescent, a mother with young children, father with young family, young adult, newborn infant, middle-aged person, the elderly and the very old. The simple philosophy that death is and will be the fate of all and that we should accept it as such clearly does not work for nurses, who are more likely than doctors to be involved intimately with the death of a patient. In this survey more than half found it very difficult to accept with equanimity the death of a young child. Moreover, sudden death evokes a different set of emotional reactions from death due to prolonged illness; for one thing, the former has been a patient for only a short time and relationships have not yet developed. The care of the terminally ill is more demanding than for other seriously ill patients, and nurses on the whole feel that the dying patient should be given priority care over others; and I suspect that other patients agree.

When the terminally ill patient brings up the topic of death and dying about half of all nurses feel relieved, a quarter uncomfortable, and the rest very uncomfortable and anxious. It is therefore important that those nursing the dying be provided with the opportunity and encouragement to talk about their patients with senior staff. No-one should be allowed to drift into the situation where he reaches an emotional or physical breaking-point unnoticed by other staff. In this regard, easy verbal communication between all nurses and all doctors pays big dividends in high morale, and aids the recognition that a break from duty is needed. The shrewd supervisor will be on the look-out for early signs of unbearable stress, and will take the appropriate action.

9

Complaints and criticism

'Anno domini – that's the most fatal complaint of all in the end.'
Mr Chips

The human mind is a wonderful organ; it works like a continuously adjustable computer. But in illness it changes: reasoning, interpretation, decision-making, previous knowledge, patience, fear and faith all become irrational. The need to concentrate effort on self-preservation takes precedence over rational thought. When people are physically ill they have a mental illness too, in the sense that the mind does not work normally. The ill patient is concerned about survival and solely interested in himself; indeed the first sign of recovery is often the patient's interest in his surroundings and other people.

Because physical illness confines normal mental agility, it is common for patients to forget what they have been told. They may misunderstand or misconstrue what they have been told. They may not accept disagreeable ideas and will defensively deny statements that were made in front of several witnesses. All this is perfectly natural. And the patient may complain.

Nobody likes to hear about grievances yet the majority are minor and easily correctable; resolving them will win the confidence and respect of the patient more quickly and more certainly than almost anything else.

Nobody likes constructive criticism; it is all we can do to put up with constructive praise. When we receive non-constructive criticism in the form of a complaint we tend to react without thinking first. On the whole doctors and nurses deal poorly with complaints because they do not appreciate what is involved.

COMMON CAUSES FOR COMPLAINTS

Grumbles and complaints are common in hospital. The vast majority are trivial, often due to misunderstanding, and could

Complaints and criticism 129

9.1 The 12 Aphorisms

1. To grumble is human.
2. Serious complaints can come from nice people.
3. All arguments about complaints have three sides: yours, mine, and the facts.
4. All complaints have some foundation.
5. Grievances grow the longer they are neglected.
6. Grievances grow in size and importance irrespective of the data.
7. A grouse becomes an official complaint with time.
8. Grievances are prolonged in proportion to the number of people involved.
9. The greater the complaint the greater the action required.
10. The majority of complaints are trivial, but it can be difficult to distinguish the trivial from the serious.
11. Prevention is better than any remedy.
12. Some complaints end up in the law courts.

be settled in seconds; too many are allowed to fester on to become major issues of discontent. James Whitcome Riley, about a century ago, wrote:

'It ain't no use to grumble and complain,
It's just as easy to rejoice;
When God sorts out the weather and sends rain
Why rain's my choice.'

which adequately sums up one attitude, but not the usual; not all complainants are quite so philosophical about their grievances. There are less trivial causes for complaints and it is as well to know how to deal with them.

The six commonest causes of complaints by patients in hospital are:

● Being given insufficient information about their condition and its management: we hear what we want to hear. We know that patients hear only about 30% of what is said in consulta-

130   *Talking with Patients*

tion; for the doctor this 'deafness' must be at least 10% and for the nurse on a busy ward even higher.

● Lack of detail of what is involved in special investigations and treatment: this lack of communication is by far the commonest foundation of all complaints.

● Pain, unrelieved and unappreciated by the attending staff.

● Noise: sometimes only the loud voice of a member of staff, but usually unexpected and unfamiliar noise within the ward (sometimes from other patients).

● The quality of food, roughness in being handled, lack of immediate attention, having to wait and being treated like a simpleton.

● No indication of the length of stay in hospital, what will happen next, when the patient can return to work; it is this uncertainty that saps morale and leads to grumbling.

All these are preventable or easily correctable, but they do require talking time from every staff member. The importance and influence of the ward sister and the junior nurses cannot be over-emphasised; they are in hourly contact with patients whereas even the most conscientious doctor cannot be. The value of a pamphlet, booklet, or even a single sheet to be given to all patients entering hospital is generally appreciated. Most hospitals now provide written information on hospital routine, hospital rules, how to obtain newspapers, books and simple toilet requisities, and who can help with personal problems of sick pay, pensions, dependents and relatives. But as Reynolds (1978) found, less than two-thirds of hospitals provide this available service.

UNDERSTANDING COMPLAINTS

What do patients do all day in hospital? Unless they are being actively treated and investigated, the choice is limited to reading the newspaper; listening to the radio; watching doctors, nurses, and other patients; and nattering with anyone who will listen. There is, therefore, an element of loneliness and boredom even in a crowded ward, which inevitably ferments complaints. And

Complaints and criticism 131

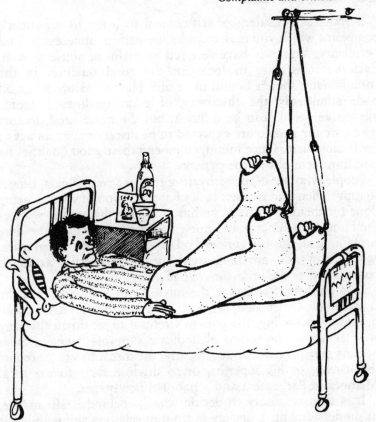

of course a complaint makes news for the visitors when they come.

So there is little wonder that patients find a need to complain, but the complaint may have a sound foundation. It is your job to find out, and find out quickly. The quarrelsome and peevish patient should be treated with circumspection. Ask yourself

Why is he so irate?
What is his main complaint?
What really has gone wrong?

If you can answer these then you are nearly half way to understanding the basis of his complaint. If you cannot, then either ask the patient outright what is wrong or defer a further confrontation until you have had time to think.

132   *Talking with Patients*

It requires considerable self-control to listen to a patient's complaint which you may consider unjustified, unnecessary and pernickity. You may have received an earful of abuse as well. Even so it is wise to look for the good qualities in the complainant; there's bound to be one. Human nature is not all bad; admittedly the discovery of good qualities in some aggressive people can be difficult, but the nurses and doctors who care for people are expected to be discerning, as an act of professionalism. Once found, commend these good qualities by pointing them out to the patient.

People who are ill, or recovering from a severe illness, do get snappy. Their bad temper, lack of appreciation of what is being done for them and loss of ambition to help themselves worries the family. The doctor and nurse will have to spend some time explaining all this to aggrieved relatives. The wife who, in tears, says 'I can't do anything right for him' deserves as much consolation as the unfortunate patient.

It is important to gauge the intensity of feeling behind the complaint. A clenched fist, the pointing index finger, hand thumping, scowling, the patient's refusal to sit down (he may wander about the room) all indicate suppressed anger. Such actions may precede (or accompany) the threat to sue, to report the listener to his superior, or to disclose facts to the local Member of Parliament and a national newspaper.

It is then necessary to decide what is behind it all: malice, misunderstanding, a display in front of relatives and mainly for their benefit, or simply a desire for equity for a social grievance? Much depends on how you interpret the complainant's actions. It is sensible to open your dialogue with the complainant by discussing the problem in general, but the details have to be faced too. All this is best sorted out in a calm atmosphere.

What does the patient expect? What can he reasonably expect from those looking after him? The list is probably endless but the eight below are important, although not necessarily listed in order of importance; the patient expects:

● confidentiality in what he says,

● a certain amount of kindness,

● decorum in the dress, behaviour and speech of the doctors and nurses as a sign of their own self-respect,

Complaints and criticism 133

● knowledge and ability to care for him, to give advice, and to help him solve problems and make decisions,

● some leadership qualities that will inspire confidence and trust, which in illness are far more important than affection; also a sense of understanding of other people,

● interest in him and his illness,

● his illness to be taken seriously, not flippantly,

● respect for him as an individual and not just as one of the herd in the hospital ward.

What does the patient hope for? Firstly, to be recognised by name because that is his individual identity which is so precious. Secondly, to be liked by members of staff. Thirdly, to be made to feel important as often as possible; at a ward round or demonstration the youngest and oldest of patients will appreciate this more than anything else.

These are not excessive expectations. Fulfilled, they are evidence of efficiency and training by doctors and nurses; unfulfilled, they are the seeds of complaints. The person who stops to chat informally and regularly with patients will rarely be the object of criticism, but he will hear complaints about other people in advance of publication and so be able to do something about them. Where there are good relationships between patients and staff there is normally a flow of information; some will be useful, some important, and the listener will have to analyse their worth.

DEALING WITH COMPLAINTS

The unit, team or hospital can choose one of two methods for dealing with complaints. One is a continuing policy of projecting an image of concern for the patient in all aspects of his illness and environment, by making all staff report every suspicion of complaint to a higher authority. By this continuous monitoring of patients, complaints can be recognised early and something done about them. Alternatively one may operate a contingent policy which reacts to trouble as and when it occurs, and which builds a technique of procedure for dealing with complaints as they arise.

134   *Talking with Patients*

The important thing is this: you cannot afford to have no policy. The best policy is probably a combination of the two, but it does demand continuous watchfulness, and there are ten points to keep in mind.

● Treat every complaint seriously and respectfully, however trivial it may seem to you. Be accessible because it is the informal method of communication that is crucial and none more so than the personal appearance and accessibility of those in charge. If patients want answers to questions, give them in person if necessary. Complaints need action, but mainly the need is to talk.

● The complaint may be expressed in fiery and abusive language, but it is vitally important never to be rude or to get heated in return. He who swears is lost, and rudeness is unprofessional conduct anyway. Keep calm and pleasant throughout. Friendliness, tact, tolerance and kindness are four important assets for the mediator. All can be cultivated and practised. Emotionalism imposes a great necessity on doctors and nurses to keep cool. There are only three possibilities: first, that what is said is true and damaging, in which case you have

---

9.2 Five steps in good management of complaints

1. The pre-approach. Learn all you can before seeing the patient. Do it now.

2. The approach. Introduce yourself. Listen to the patient. Ask questions. Write notes.

3. The presentation. Summarise what the patient has said and your interpretation in simple clear language. Be objective.

4. Dealing with the complaint. Investigate in detail. Discover the facts and the solutions.

5. The close. Discuss what can be done. Allow the patient to decide on the plan of action. Ask if he is satisfied. Express gratitude for drawing your attention to a complaint which will not be mentioned again.

Complaints and criticism 135

to correct the fault immediately; second, that what is said is false and damaging in which case you can sue; third, that what is said, whether true or false, is not damaging so why not make friends rather than enemies? Undoubtedly the person who persistently shuns confrontation communicates a vital and destructive message: fear.

● Treat complaints as emergencies, to be dealt with expeditiously. Try to deal with the complaint that day if at all possible and say that you will return later, at a specific time, to report progress rather than defer action until tomorrow.

● Never argue, if only because no battle is won by argument. The only way to get the best of an argument is to avoid it. You can avoid all arguments by explaining that you will investigate fully and report back to the patient. You can use 'but' as a form of temporary delay as with 'the nurses are busy, but I will find out'.

● Listen to the patient attentively. Let him do most of the talking, but ask questions for clarification, then summarise in your own words if the complaint is not clear in your own mind.

● Investigate the complaint, by questioning others and do some foot-work if necessary. You may have to sit down and try to analyse the reasons for the complaint before doing anything about it; five minutes' contemplation is often invaluable, to get at the core of the matter.

Try to understand the patient's position, especially in hospital. He is bed-bound in a strange environment, not feeling too good, wholly dependent on those who serve him, his precious pills confiscated, and he may be lonely, depressed and frightened.

● If you are in the wrong, say so. You can explain how things went wrong and if the patient is not satisfied do offer to provide a second opinion. Remember to apologise, but the apology must come after the complaint has been looked into. Make your explanation brief and to the point, so tell the truth and act accordingly, and you cannot go wrong. The liar is doubly damaged: by the truth he sought to disguise, and by its exposure when the truth escapes.

● If the complaint is not directly your responsibility, say so

136 *Talking with Patients*

and tell the patient that you will find out who is responsible and report back later in the day (or next morning, but try to give an indication of the time). Do make the most of the opportunity and take the initiative in soothing bruised feelings on both sides (the aggrieved and the aggressor) and thank the patient for drawing your attention to the complaint. Better still, say that you will return in two days to ask if the patient is satisfied that the complaint has been dealt with adequately, because you too are interested in the outcome. This is a form of flattery that few can resist. It usually takes the heat out of a grave situation and can turn the trivial into the humorous. Moreover, it implies that the complaint will be analysed with the greatest care to discover what the real grievance is, and that there will be a full and fair response.

● Do point out the patient's right to complain and the procedure for making an official complaint. In hospital the ward sister is responsible for the day-to-day running of a ward; she usually tours her territory once a day, and should be the first to hear of any complaint. If there is good rapport, the doctor in charge of the patient will be alerted immediately and can do something quickly. For serious complaints it is my practice to see the patient with a hospital administrator, explaining that the

---

9.3 Faults in dealing with complaints

1. Not listening to the complainant.
2. Not clarifying the complaint.
3. Getting bogged down in trivia.
4. Failing to show sympathy.
5. Neglecting to explain why and how.
6. Blaming others.
7. Apologising too soon.
8. Doing nothing.
9. Absolute denial.
10. The cover-up.

Complaints and criticism 137

latter is there so that the patient can make his complaint official and that it will be reported to the appropriate health authority if the patient so desires; very few patients pursue the matter further, but some do, so write in the records at the time any details that may be required later.

● Remember to thank the patient for bringing the complaint to your attention. There should be no stigma attached to any patient with a genuine complaint and it is your duty to make sure that the patient is not labelled uncooperative. The Royal College of Nursing conducted a survey into the unpopular patient in 1974 and found that such people received considerably worse care in hospital than popular patients who talked readily to nurses, knew their names, and never complained. Such behaviour is understandable, but inexcusable.

For the effective trouble-shooter, two things matter more than anything else: reputation and reliability. The reputation for fairness, action, firmness, discipline, and for always being on the spot at the right time or readily available. These alone guarantee patient satisfaction.

The basis of good morale in patients is undoubtedly the easy and free flow of information by word of mouth. What begins as a routine becomes a habit, a practised habit becomes a skill, and a skill develops self-confidence. By overcoming reluctance to talk with patients we learn self-discipline, and by talking we learn to talk, which is self-achievement. 'If a man would move the world, he must first move himself' (Paul).

References and further reading

The best way to be in a position to judge issues is to read around them. There are three basic types of reading.

1. General textbooks on the art of communicating with patients.
2. Specialised reading which may go into greater depth than you need. It is often necessary to confine reading to some of the chapters; for instance, in books on speech training, voice production, drama, general medicine, nursing and so on. So browse among the library shelves.
3. Journals often contain articles on listening and talking, organisation of hospital wards and waiting rooms, and related subjects. Look for such papers in the *British Medical Journal, Lancet, Science, Journal of Medical Education, New England Journal of Medicine, Journal of the American Medical Association*, and several others. Photocopy or make notes from the most helpful papers, and so build up your own file of references.

Abercrombie M.L.J. (1972). Non-verbal communication. *Proceedings of the Royal Society of Medicine*; 65: 335–6.

Anderson J., Day J.L., Dowling M.A.C., Pettingale K.W. (1970). The definition and evaluation of skill required to obtain a patient's history of illness: the use of videotape recordings. *Postgraduate Medical Journal*; 46: 606–12.

Anderson D., Ward V. (1979). *English Tests for Doctors*. London: Nelson.

Apley V. (1980). Communicating with children. *British Medical Journal*; 281: 1116–7.

Ashe G. (1979). *The Art of Writing, Made Simple*. London: Allen.

Asher R.A.J. (1959). Making sense. *Lancet*; ii: 359–65.

Asher R.A.J. (1972). Richard Asher talking sense. *The Sir Francis Avery Jones Edition of Collected Papers*. London: Pitman Medical.

Balint M. (1957). *The Doctor, his Patient and the Illness*. (2nd edn) London: Pitman.

References and further reading 139

Balint M. (1964). The doctor's therapeutic function. *Lancet*; i: 1177–80.

Barber, G. (1966). Communication in medicine. *Practitioner*; **196**: 134–8.

Bennett A.E., ed (1976). *Communication between Doctors and Patients*. Nuffield Provincial Hospitals Trust. London: Oxford University Press.

Bennett G. (1974). Scientific medicine? *Lancet*; ii: 453–6.

Bennett G. (1979) *Patients and their Doctors*. London: Balliére Tindall.

Boyle C.M. (1970). Differences between patients' and doctors' interpretation of some common medical terms. *British Medical Journal*; **2**: 286–9.

Brewin T.B. (1977). The cancer patient: communication and morale. *British Medical Journal*; **3**: 1623–7.

Burkinshaw K. (1977). But I do want to know. *World Medicine*; May 18: 88.

Byrne P.S., Long B.E. (1976). *Doctors Talking to Patients*. London: HMSO.

Calnan J., Barabas A. (1981). *Speaking at Medical Meetings: a Practical Guide*, 2nd edn. London: William Heinemann Medical Books.

Cargill D. (1968). Communication between doctors and patients. *Proceedings of the Royal Society of Medicine*; **61**: 563–5.

Cartwright A. (1964), *Human Relations and Hospital Care*. London: Routledge and Kegan Paul.

Central Health Services Council. (1963). *Communication between Doctors, Nurses and Patients: An Aspect of Human Relations in the Hospital Service*. London: HMSO.

Christman L.P. (1965). Nurse–physician communication in the hospital. *Journal of the American Medical Association*; **194**: 539–44.

140 *Talking with Patients*

Cheyney P.S. (1980). ed. Nursing Skillbook Series No. 78. *Dealing with Death and Dying*, 2nd edn. Intermed Communications, Horsham, Pa.

Cochrane A.L. (1971). *Effectiveness and Efficiency*. (Rock Carling Lecture 1970). Nuffield Provincial Hospitals Trust. London: Oxford University Press.

Cochrane A.L. (1976). Some reflections. In *A question of quality?* (McLachlan G., ed.) p. 259. Nuffield Provincial Hospitals Trust. London: Oxford University Press.

Cousins N. (1976). The Anatomy of an illness as perceived by the patient. *New England Journal of Medicine*; 295: 1458–63.

Crystal D. (1971). *Linguistics*. Harmondsworth: Penguin.

Diamond A.S. (1959). *The History and Origin of Language*. London: Methuen.

Dirckx J.H. (1976). *The Language of Medicine: Evolution, Structure and Dynamics*. New York: Harper and Row.

Drucker P. (1975). *The Practice of Management*. London: Heinemann.

Duncan A.S., Dunstan G.R., Welbourn R.B., eds. (1981). *The Dictionary of Medical Ethics*, 2nd edn. Darton, Longman and Todd.

Dunkelman H. (1979). Patient's knowledge of their condition and treatment: how it might be improved. *British Medical Journal*; 3: 311–14.

Egbert L.D., Battit G.E., Welch C.E., Bartlett M.K. (1964). Reduction of post-operative pain by encouragement and instruction of patients. *New England Journal of Medicine*; 270: 825–7.

Fletcher C.M. (1968). Communication between doctors and patients. *Proceedings of the Royal Society of Medicine*; 61: 567–8.

Fletcher C.M (1973). *Communication in Medicine*. (The Rock Carling Fellowship 1972). The Nuffield Provincial Hospitals Trust. London: Oxford University Press.

References and further reading 141

Fletcher C.M. (1979). In *Mixed Communication: Essays on Current Research*. Nuffield Provincial Hospitals Trust. London: Oxford University Press.

Fletcher C.M. (1980). Listening and talking to patients. *British Medical Journal*; 4: 845–7, 931–3, 994–6, 1056–8.

Fowler H.W., Fowler F.G. (1962). *The King's English*, 3rd edn. Oxford: Clarendon Press.

Fox T.F. (1965). *Crisis in Communication*. London: Athlone Press.

Gimson A.C. (1970). *An Introduction to the Pronunciation of English*, 2nd edn. London: Edward Arnold.

Gowers E. (1973). *The Complete Plain Words*, 2nd edn. revised by Sir Bruce Fraser. London: HMSO.

Hawkins C.F. (1967). *Speaking and Writing in Medicine*. USA: Thomas, Springfield.

Hawkins C. (1979). Patients' reactions to their investigations: a study of 504 patients. *British Medical Journal*; 2: 638–40.

Herxheimer A. (1977). Keep on taking the tablets. *British Medical Journal*; 1: 974.

Herzberg F. (1966). *Work and the Nature of Man*. Cleveland, USA: World Publishing.

Hinton J. (1972). *Dying*, 2nd edn. Harmondsworth: Penguin.

Hinton J. (1980s). Whom do dying patients tell? *British Medical Journal*; 4: 1328–30.

Jagger J.H. (1960). *A Handbook of English Grammar*. London: University of London Press.

Joss M. (1967). *The Five Clocks*. New York: Harcourt.

Kubler-Ross E. (1969). *On Death and Dying*. London: Macmillan.

Ley P. (1973). The measurement of comprehensibility. *Journal of Institute of Health Education*; 11: 17–20.

142 Talking with Patients

Ley P. (1977). Psychological studies of doctor patient communication. In *Contributiions to Medical Psychology* (Rachman S., ed.) Oxford: Pergamon Press.

McColl I., Drinkwater J.E., Hume-Moir I., Donnan S.R.B. (1971). Predicting success or failure of gastric surgery. *British Journal of Surgery*; 58: 768–71.

McGregor D. (1960). *The Human Side of Enterprise.* New York: McGraw-Hill.

Maslow A.H. (1954). *Motivation and Personality.* New York: Harper & Row.

Meadows A.J. (1974). *Communication in Science.* London: Butterworth.

Meares A. (1954). Rapport with the patient, symbolic significance of the doctor's behaviour. *Lancet*; ii: 592–4.

Melmon K.L., Grossman M., Morris R.C. (1970). Emerging assets and liabilities of a committee on human welfare and experimentation. *New England Journal of Medicine*; 282: 427–31.

Miller G.E., Graser H.P., Abrahamson S., Harnack R.S., Cohen I.S., Land A. (1962). *Teaching and Learning in Medical School.* The Commonwealth Fund. Mass: Harvard University Press.

Moll J.M.H., Wright V. (1978). *Communicating with the Patient.* Reports on Rheumatic Diseases No. 64. (Hawkins C., Currey HL.F., eds.) London: The Arthritis and Rheumatism Council.

Morris D. (1977). *Manwatching. A Field-guide to Human Behaviour.* London: Jonathan Cape.

Morris D., Collett P., Marsh P., O'Shaughnessy M. (1979). *Gestures: their Orgins and Distributions.* London: Jonathan Cape.

Murphy F., Bentley S., Ellis B.W., Dudley H. (1977). Sleep deprivation in patients undergoing operation: a factor in the stress of surgery. *British Medical Journal*; 4: 1521–2.

Nathan P.C., Barrowclough A.R. (1957). *Medical Negligence.* London: Butterworth.

References and further reading   143

Neill J. (1968). Communication between doctors and patients. *Proceedings of the Royal Society of Medicine*; **61**: 565–7.

Newman A.D., Summer B. (1961). *The Process of Management*. New Jersey: Prentice-Hall.

Nuffield Working Party on Communication with Patients (1980). *Talking with Patients: A Teaching Approach*. London: Nuffield Provincial Hospitals Trust. (Includes, at the end, a useful reading list by Professor Fletcher.)

Pappworth M.H. (1978). Medical ethical committees: a review of their functions. *World Medicine*, 22 February; p. 69 onwards.

Parkinson J.E. (1971). *A Manual of English for the Overseas Doctor*. Edinburgh: Churchill Livingstone.

Parkinson J.E. (1978). *English for Doctors and Nurses*. London: Evans Brothers.

Partridge E. (1978). *Usage and Abusage: a Guide to Good English*, 6th edn. London: Hamish Hamilton.

Pearson J., Dudley H.A.F. (1982). Bodily perceptions in surgical patients. *British Medical Journal*; **284**: 1545–6.

Pickering G. (1961). Language, the last tool of learning in medicine and science. *Lancet*; **ii**: 115–9.

Price J.I.W. (1977). The patient's morale. *Lancet*; **1**: 533.

Querido A. (1959). Forecast and follow-up: An investigation into the clinical, social and mental factors determining the results of hospital treatment. *British Journal of Preventive and Social Medicine*; **13**: 33–49.

Reynolds M. (1978). No news is bad news: patients' views about communication in hospital. *British Medical Journal*; **1**: 1673–6.

Saunders C., ed. (1978). *The Management of Terminal Disease*. London: Edward Arnold.

Scadding J.G. (1967). Diagnosis: the clinician and the computer. *Lancet*; **ii**: 877–81.

144 Talking with Patients

Stimson G., Webb B. (1975). *Going to See the Doctor*. London: Routledge and Kegan Paul.

Stork E.C., Widdowson J.D.A. (1974). *Learning about Linguistics*. London: Hutchinson.

Taggart P., Carruthers M., Somerville W. (1973). Electrocardiograms, plasma catecholamines and lipids and their modification by oxyprenolol when speaking before an audience. *Lancet*; ii: 341–6.

Thomson R.D., Irvine A.H. (1960). *Everyday English Usage*. London: Collins.

Tanner B.A., ed. (1976). *Language and Communication in General Practice*. London: Hodder & Stoughton.

Van Hooff J. (1962). Facial expressions in higher primates. *Symposia Zoological Society of London*; 8: 97–125.

Wallechinsky D., Wallace I., Wallace A. (1977). *The Book of Lists*. London: Cassell.

Wells G. (1978). *How to communicate*. London: McGraw-Hill.

Wild A.A., Evans J. (1968). The patient and the x-ray department. *British Medical Journal*; 2: 607–9.

Wilkinson A., Statta L., Dudley P. (1974). *The Quality of Listening*. London: Methuen.

Wilson J.B. (1961). Doctor and patient today. *Lancet*; ii: 201–2.

Wilson-Barnett J. (1979). *Stress in Hospital*. Edinburgh: Churchill Livingstone.

Index

*References are made to nurses, doctors and patients on most pages
and are not listed specifically here.*

Abilities, six important, 11
Ability, 1, 30, 36, 105, 111,
    124, 133
Actor, 9
Advantages, to patient, 17,
    30, 92, 115
Advice, 22, 77, 102, 103, 106,
    121, 133
Affectation, 45
Affection, 36, 124, 133
Aggrieved, 128
Aim
    conversation, of, 35
    interview, of, 49
Anaesthetist, 77, 102, 106
Analysis, 12, 50, 54, 58, 78,
    82, 135
Anatomy, 102
Anonymous, 107
Answers, 10, 108, 134
    need for, 60
Aphorisms, the twelve, 129
Argument, 40, 92, 120, 135
Art, 9
    interview, of, 49
    listening, of, 57
    persuasion, of, 79
Attitude(s), 2, 17, 20, 22,
    26, 27, 35, 38, 55, 89,
    115
    doctor/nurse, of, 2, 46, 67,
    80

    patient, of, 17, 30, 36, 119,
    121, 129
Audio-visual, 12
Authority, 7, 9, 87, 90, 105,
    119, 124
Awareness, 3

Bereaved, 124
Bereavement, 89, 111, 125
Blind, the, 63, 64
Boredom, 34, 130
Bravery, 116

C's, the three, 105
C's, the four, 124
Cancer, 83, 111
Care, 11, 93, 105, 114, 125,
    132, 137
Causes
    complaints, of, 128, 129
    disease, of, 81
Charisma, 6
Chat, 32, 106, 121
Check list, 101
Children, 63, 82, 89, 96, 98,
    109, 123
    parents, and, 66
Clarity, 21
Clinical trials, 74, 76
Comfort, 9, 39, 69, 85, 113,
    122, 124, 125
Commitment, 38, 124

146　*Talking with Patients*

Communication, 1, 5, 7, 9,
　58, 97, 108, 116, 118,
　126, 130, 134
　patient, and the, 27
　significance of, 30
　twelve principles, 14
Competence, 30
Complaints, 42, 78, 128, 133
　causes of, 128, 129
　faults in dealing with, 134,
　　136
　how to deal with, 133, 134
　managing, 134
　understanding, 130, 132
Compliance, 95, 97, 99
Complications, 61, 79, 104
Concept, 16, 100, 103, 111
Conclusions
　diagnosis, of, 84
　interview, of, 49, 51
Confidence, 9, 12, 27, 30,
　118, 119, 123, 124, 128
Confidential, 28, 51, 53, 54,
　69, 71, 132
Connotations, of words, 14,
　62, 71, 74, 82, 94, 109
Consent
　forms, 76, 102
　informed, 74, 75, 76, 77,
　　78, 79, 101
Consequences of diagnosis, 85
Consultation
　skill of, 22
　technique, 35, 53, 82
Contact, physical, 10, 124
Control, 34, 51, 74
　span of, 118
Conversation, 9, 27, 32, 38,
　39, 41, 57, 59, 87, 93,
　107, 110, 116
　principles, 34

Counselling, 55, 125
Courage, 73, 84, 116, 124
Courtesy, 30, 41, 105, 106,
　117
Criticism, 123, 133
Cure, 11, 81, 100, 111, 115

D's, the four, 117
Deaf, 28, 29, 63, 109
Dealing with complaints, 133,
　134
Death
　peaceful, 116
　talking of, 61, 69, 88, 111,
　　113, 116, 124, 126
Decision making, 77, 78, 95,
　128
Decisions, 11, 16, 27, 30, 48,
　77, 104
Definition
　communication, of, 14
　consent, of, 76
　consultation, of, 48
　conversation, of, 32
　diagnosis, of, 81
Deformity, 79, 88
Deftness, 11
Delegate, 11, 31, 116
Demand, 80, 91, 120
Demonstration, 72, 133
Demonstrator, 72
Details, 108
Diagnosis
　attitude of patient to, 119
　explaining, 7, 36, 41, 52,
　　58, 60, 66, 68, 77, 82, 93
　guides to, 83, 101, 103
　types of, 81
　why patient must know, 85
Diagrams, 84, 103
Dialogue, 33, 48, 132

Index 147

Disability, 37, 61, 63, 79, 88, 89
Disadvantages of bad communication, 30, 92, 115
Disbeliever, 121
Discharge, from hospital, 73, 77, 106
Discomfort, 79, 108
Discussion, 50, 58, 68, 72, 74
Disfigurement, 61, 79, 88
Disposables, 99
Donor organs, 77, 79
Drugs
  compliance, 100
  information, 101, 115
  side effects, 61, 100
Duty
  demonstrator, of, 72
  patient, to, 73, 112, 116, 121
Dying, 69, 112, 113

Effective communication, 5, 17, 24, 28
Emergency, 78, 108, 135
Emotions, 3, 14, 21, 26, 46, 113
  stages of, 67, 119
Empathy, 6, 22
Encode, 26
Encouragement, 54, 66, 96, 126
English, 7, 12, 25, 71, 112
Enjoyment, 12, 33
Enthusiasm, 43
Environment, 8, 20, 46, 96, 108, 123, 133, 135
Ethical Committee, 74, 75
Ethics, 10, 75
Etiquette, 75

Evidence, 77, 90, 106, 121
Expectation, 24, 91, 93, 94, 115, 133
Experience, 3, 14, 24, 41, 72, 87
Expertise, 124
Explanation
  patient, to, 80, 81, 85, 97, 102, 108, 120
  technique, 84, 90, 93
Expressions, 22, 71

Fatal illness, 67, 87, 111, 115, 120
Favoured treatment, 122
Fear, 28, 44, 53, 59, 67, 84, 88, 90, 91, 114, 117, 119, 121, 128, 135
  groups, 106
  hidden, 122
Feed back, 19, 20, 23, 25, 26, 29, 34, 43
Foreigners, 63, 69
Forms
  consent, of, 76, 102
  instructions, of, 64, 66, 98, 101, 102, 109
  talking, of, 4
Foundation, to complaints, 131
Friendliness, 27, 36, 44, 51, 87, 124, 134

Gesture(s), 22, 27, 34, 35, 59, 64, 124
  communication, 18, 19, 21, 70
  mimicry, 21, 26, 70
  non-verbal/non-vocal, 21, 45
Greeting, 51, 53, 63, 65

148　*Talking with Patients*

Grieve, 69, 125
Guilt, 69, 112

Handshake, 27, 53, 54, 65, 66
Harassed, 122
Helpless, 122
Honesty, 117
Hope, 60, 83
Hopeless, 88, 122
Hospice, 113, 118, 126
Hospital, 7
Humour, 6, 91, 112, 124
　conversation, in, 33, 43
　use of, 44
　value of, 44

Ignorance, 115, 116
Illustrations, 12, 18, 22, 27, 70, 103, 118
Improvement, in talking, 7
Inference, 18, 20
Information, 10, 16, 17, 23, 26, 34, 38, 41, 114
Instructions, 64, 66, 98, 101, 102, 109
Integrity, 7, 12
Interference, 25
Interpretation, 20
　interview, of, 54
　investigations, of, 110
Interpreter, 34, 71
Interview, 35, 48, 84
　aim of, 49
　length of, 113
　skills, 49, 53
　success, 52
Introductions, 68, 73
Investigations, 36, 51, 52, 60, 76, 86, 90, 93, 101, 110, 122, 130

Jargon, 70, 84
Joke, 44
Judgement, 12, 57, 87

Kindness, 11, 43, 68, 69, 110, 132, 134
Knack, 11, 46
Knowledge, 5, 41, 87
　current, 42
　lacking, 36

Language, 7, 18, 21, 25, 28, 34, 41, 65, 99, 103, 109, 114
Leadership, 12, 30, 133
Lecture, 33, 100, 110
Lip-read, 63, 65
Listen, 27, 116
　how to, 57, 58, 135
Listening, 24, 27, 28, 37, 47, 53, 121
Litigation, 80, 104
Logic, 17, 51
Loneliness, 38, 67, 113, 114, 123, 130
Love, 36, 43, 113

Management, of patient, 41, 61, 74, 87, 95, 102, 123, 129, 134
Mannerisms, 45, 46
Manners, 45, 53, 74, 86
Medicine, talking, 40, 49
Meetings, 72
Message, 14, 17, 23, 28, 29,
Mimicry, 21, 26, 70 38
Monologue, 33, 34, 66
Morale, 10, 30, 44, 106, 124, 127, 130, 137

Need, 96

Index 149

Noise, 25, 64, 109, 130
Non-compliance, 97
Non-verbal/non-vocal, 20, 26, 45
  communication, 21

Operation
  investigation, 102
  surgical, 61, 78, 79, 101, 102, 105
Opinion, second, 72, 80, 86, 105, 135
Optimist, 90, 120

Pain, 67, 69, 74, 79, 83, 88, 105, 106, 107, 108, 113, 125, 130
Palliation, 100
Pamphlet, 130
Parents, 66, 82, 123
Participation, 5, 102
Passive patient, 122
Pattern, 20
Pauses, 34, 64, 71, 112
  use of, 43
Perception, 3, 15, 17, 20, 42, 57, 125
Perfection, 28
Performance, 5, 72, 118
Permission, 72, 79, 118
Perspective, 36
Persuasion, 5, 16, 29, 50, 79, 80, 95
Pharmacy, 98
Philosophical, 120
Photographs, 103
Place, of interview, 48, 52
Planning, of talk, 33
Politeness, 30
Post-mortem, 77, 79
Praise, 37

Predictions, 88, 89
Preliminaries, to communication, 16
Preparation
  interview, for, 50
  talking, for, 122
Preventive, 36
Principles
  communication, of, 5, 28
  conversation, of, 33
  performance, and, 5
Privacy, 51, 52, 68, 91, 107, 111, 113, 117
Privilege, 9
Problem, 12, 50, 89, 112, 123, 133
Professionalism, 6, 7, 132
Prognosis, 10, 87, 93
  prediction, 88
Progress, 42, 62, 75
Prompt sheet, 100
Provocation, 12
Purpose
  communication, of, 15, 16, 24, 110
  conversation, of, 38
  interview, of, 48, 52, 73

Questionnaire, 23, 50
Questions, 2, 10, 28, 36, 49, 53, 77, 84, 102, 106, 134
  compliance, about, 100
  drug actions, of, 100
  skill of, 55
  types of, 55
  uses of, 55

Rapport, 35, 53, 54
Reassurance, 10, 36, 61, 89, 119

150   *Talking with Patients*

Recipient, of communication, 14, 24
Records, 49, 54, 86, 101, 105, 137
Recovery, 106
References, 138
Relationships, 2, 17, 32, 33, 35, 38, 42, 73, 105, 114, 116
Relatives, of patient, 52, 60, 65, 67, 76, 105, 113, 122 132
Remembering, 22, 38, 67, 100, 102
Repetition, 17, 26, 58, 64, 84, 94, 99
Reprimand, 11
Research, 42, 74, 115
   description, 75
   explanation, 75
Respect, 3, 6, 41, 73, 83, 99, 110, 128, 133
Responsibility, 12, 73, 96
Rhythm, of speaking, 19, 34, 58, 112
Rights, of patient, 136
Risks, 76, 82, 90, 104

Salesmanship, 5, 92
Scars, 104
Scientific method, 81, 82
Secrecy, 69, 76, 84
Seminar, 72
Side-effects, 61, 97, 100, 121
Signals, 26, 34
Skill, 3, 4, 6, 28, 123, 137
   conversation, of, 37
   interview, of, 84
Sleep, 10, 107
Smell, 27
Smile, 2, 27, 37, 43, 53, 59, 63

Social background, 22, 89
Sources, of information, 114
Speaker, attractive, 112
Speaking, 17, 66
Speechless, the, 65
Speed, of communication, 20, 25
Spiritual, 11, 113
Spoken communication, 14, 19
Staff, talking with, 41, 126
Stages
   communication, of, 16
   grief, of, 67, 119
Stigma, 137
Stimulation, 20, 39, 108
Strain, 107
Stress, of talking, 3
Stripping, 107
Structure
   conversation, of, 32, 34
   interview, of, 32, 51
Struggle, 107
Style, 2, 41, 42, 46, 112
Surgeon, 77, 102, 105, 109
Survival, 107, 113
Suspicious, 2, 53, 90, 121

Tact, 4, 80, 114, 117, 134
Talent, 2
Talker, the good, 6, 111
Talking, 11, 42, 114
   bereaved, with, 124
   death, of, 117
   faults in, 71
   medical, 40, 49
   planning, 114
   reasons for, 39, 114
   relatives, with, 67
   staff, with, 126
   stress, 3

Index 151

Teaching, on patients, 72
  talking, 2
Techniques, of talking, 1
Terminal illness, 10, 125
Tests, 36, 82, 122, 126
Time, to talk, 16, 29, 48, 56,
  110
Tolerance, 33, 39, 43,
  134
Touch, 2, 27, 65, 124
Training, 111, 113
Treatment, 41, 58, 68, 80, 86,
  95, 103, 130
Trust, 12, 27, 28, 30, 35, 49,
  51, 71, 108, 109, 111,
  118, 123, 133
Truth, 10, 115, 135
Types, of conversation, 39

Understanding, 23, 28, 42, 88,
  95, 101, 106, 118
  communication, 5, 9, 12,
  15, 19
  complaints, 130

Value, 17, 23, 35, 56, 90, 96,
  117
Visitors, 72, 118
Visual communication, 18
Vocabulary, 12, 19, 23, 33, 40
Vocation, 11

Ward round, 10, 42, 72, 105,
  123, 133
Welcome, 51, 53, 109
Words, 22, 35, 88, 116
  connotations, 14, 62, 71,
  74, 82, 94, 109
  right, 26, 46, 61, 66
Work, 36
Worry, 33, 36, 37, 38, 59, 68,
  81, 98, 106, 121, 123,
  132
Writers, 91
Writing, 27, 58, 64, 101, 103
Written communication, 17,
  23, 98, 102, 117

X-rays, 51, 110